CURRENT RESEARCH ON SUICIDE AND PARASUICIDE

CURRENT RESEARCH ON SUICIDE AND PARASUICIDE

Selected proceedings of the Second European Symposium on Suicidal Behaviour, Edinburgh, June 1988

Edited by
Stephen David Platt and Norman Kreitman

Edinburgh University Press

22 George Square, Edinburgh

Set in Lasercomp Century Schoolbook
and printed in Great Britain by
The Alden Press Ltd
London and Oxford

British Library Cataloguing
in Pulication Data
European Symposium on Suicidal Behaviour: 2nd (1988)
Current research on suicide and parasuicide: selected
proceedings of the Second European Symposium on
Suicidal Behaviour.
1. Suicide. Psychosocial aspects
I. Title II. Kreitman, Norman III. Platt, Stephen
David
362.2

ISBN 0 85224 629 3

CONTENTS

LIST OF CONTRIBUTORS

BANON, D. Department of Psychiatry, University of Padua.
BARTH, P. Department of Psychiatry I, University of Ulm.
BELL, V. Department of Psychiatry II, University of Ulm, Gunzburg Hospital.
BLUMENTHAL, St. Department of Psychiatry II, University of Ulm, Gunzburg Hospital.
CLEIREN, M.P.H.D. Department of Clinical Psychology, University of Leiden.
COSTA, G. Epidemiologist, Torino.
CREPET, P. Psychiatrist and Sociologist, National Research Centre, Rome.
DALY, M. Consultant Psychiatrist, St Anne's Hospital, Shanakiel, Cork.
DEISTER, A. Psychiatric Department, University of Bonn.
DIEKSTRA, R.F.W. Division of Mental Health, World Health Organisation, Geneva.
DIETZFELBINGER, T. Psychiatric Clinic, University of Munich.
FLORENZANO, F. Psychologist, Rome.
FLURSCHUTZ, E. Psychiatric Clinic, Bad Hersfield, West Germany.
GAUTIER, J.Y. Psychiatrist, Charcot Hospital, Caudaon.
HARMAT, P. Department of Neurology and Psychology, Linz General Hospital.
HAWTON, K. Department of Psychiatry, University of Oxford.
HEIM, N. Institute of Social Medicine, Free University of Berlin.
HOLE, G. Department of Psychiatry I, University of Ulm.
KELLEHER, M.J. Clinical Director, St Anne's Hospital, Shanakiel, Cork.

KELLER, F. Department of Psychiatry I, University of Ulm.
KEOHANE, L.B. Social Worker, St Anne's Hospital, Shanakiel, Cork.
KERKHOF, A.J.F.M. Department of Clinical Health and Personality Psychology, University of Leiden.
KURZ, A. Psychiatric Clinic, University of Munich.
DE LEO, D. Department of Psychiatry, University of Padua.
LINEHAN, C. Social Research.
LORENZ, W. Lecturer in Social Work, University College, Cork.
MARNEROS, A. Department of Psychiatry, University of Bonn.
MEIER, G. Max-Planck-Institute for Psychology, Munich.
MOESLER, T.A. Psychiatry Division, University of Erlangen-Nuremburg.
MOLLER, H.J. Professor, Psychiatric Clinic, University of Munich.
MORITZ, B.J.M. Department of Clinical and Health Psychology, Unviersity of Leiden.
NEUMANN, N.-U. Department of Psychiatry II, University of Ulm.
PAVAN, L. Department of Psychiatry, University of Padua.
PENQUIL, F. Centre Anti-Poison, Bordeaux.
PHILIPPE, A. National Institute of Health and Medical Research, Le Vesinet.
POMMEREAU, X. Hospital Centre, University of Bordeaux.
ROHDE, A. Department of Psychiatry, University of Bonn.
SCHALLER, S. Otto-Seiz Institute, University of Mannheim.
SCHIFAND, F. Department of Psychiatry, University of Padua.
SCHMIDTKE, A. Department of Psychiatry, University of Wuerzburg.
SCHUTTLER, R. Professor of Psychiatry, University of Ulm, Gunzburg Psychiatric Hospital.
STEINER, B. Department of Psychiatry II, University of Ulm.
TEDO, P. Jean Sarrailh Centre, Aire-sur-Adour.
TORHORST, A. Psychiatric Clinic, University of Munich.
TRICOT, L. Department of Psychiatry, University of Geneva.
VASCON, M. Department of Psychiatry, University of Padua.
VERRON, M. Research Assistant, National Institute of Health and Medical Research.
VISSER, A.P. Social Psychologist, Faculty of Health Sciences, State University of Limberg. Le Vesinet.

VOGEL, R. Department of Psychiatry II, University of Ulm, Gunzburg Psychiatric Hospital.

WAL, VAN DER, J. Department of Clinical and Health Psychology, University of Leiden.

WEIDENHAMMER, W. Psychiatry Division, University of Erlangen-Nuremburg.

WOLFERSDORF, M. Department of Psychiatry I, University of Ulm.

ZUMBRUNNEN, R. Department of Psychiatry, University of Geneva.

PREFACE

The Second European Symposium on Suicidal Behaviour was held in Edinburgh in June 1988. Over 130 speakers participated, mostly drawn from research centres in Europe, but with some distinguished contributors from North America.

The Symposium agreed, notwithstanding the general scientific excellence of the presentations, that it would not be useful to seek publication of all the papers given, since some of the work reported was destined to appear in the professional press. Accordingly, several contributors refrained from submitting their papers for consideration, but all the same many more submissions were received than could be accommodated. The editors therefore had to make many difficult, even invidious, choices and to exclude several excellent papers; inevitably the final selection is necessarily somewhat arbitrary. Nevertheless the reader has the opportunity of enjoying a unique collection of papers, which provides an overview of some of the major contemporary innovations in parasuicide and suicide research.

We take this opportunity to thank the many colleagues who helped to make the Conference so successful and to acknowledge the assistance of Royal Bank of Scotland, Marks & Spencer plc, The Scotch Whisky Association, Duphar Laboratories Ltd., and the City of Edinburgh.

N. KREITMAN
S.D. PLATT

1

NATIONAL AND INTERNATIONAL TRENDS IN SUICIDE

An international perspective on suicide and its prevention[1]

R.F.W. DIEKSTRA

Introduction

There are large international variations in death rates from suicides between the countries[2] in the world. Of those countries which report to the World Health Organization (WHO) and whose suicide rates are published in the 1987 WHO Health Statistics Annual (WHO, 1987) or are available in the WHO databank for at least one year after 1979, the range in suicide rates spans from practically zero (where are are no deaths from suicide) in countries including Malta and Egypt, to the remarkably high rate of nearly 1,000 per million on the Falkland Islands (see Table 1). The highest single yearly rate for the latest year for which data are available was for 20–24-year-old males on the Falkland Islands, at the rate of 5000 suicides per million population.[3] An inspection of Table 1 shows a pattern in the suicide rates. Arabic countries have relatively low rates of suicide. The same holds true for the Latin American countries, which also tend to have lower rates. The European countries and countries populated in the majority by people of European descent, such as Australia, the United States of America and Canada, tend to have relatively high rates. Within the European countries there is a discernible pattern also. Southern European countries have relatively low rates, while Northern and Middle European countries usually have higher rates of suicide. The Asians have rates more evenly distributed across the range. It would, however, be unjustified to consider Table 1 as a totally accurate or complete reflection of the international mortality by suicide. First of all, only seventy-one countries are reported here (some of them not being nations in the legal sense of the word) of the 166 member states of WHO today.

TABLE 1: Suicide rates in countries reporting to WHO[a] (per million of population)

Country	Males	Females	Country	Males	Females
Falklands/Maldives	1000	—	Trinidad & Tobago	121	50
Hungary	661	259	Italy	110	43
Surinam	436	128	Chile	107	18
Finland	430	113	Argentina	105	34
Austria	421	158	Ireland	92	39
Sri Lanka	377	197	Venezuela	76	20
Denmark	351	206	Israel	75	35
France	331	127	Costa Rica	74	15
Switzerland	330	132	Thailand	69	62
Belgium	326	153	Spain	68	23
Czechoslovakia	292	92	Greece	57	25
Japan	278	149	Ecuador	55	36
Fed. Rep. Germany	266	12	Cape Verde	44	6
Sweden	250	115	Martinique	44	13
Bulgaria	232	94	Bahrain	40	6
Yugoslavia	228	97	Mauritius	40	16
Poland	220	44	Paraguay	33	15
Norway	208	74	Dominica	28	—
Luxembourg	207	74	Mexico	25	7
Iceland	206	58	Barbados	25	15
Canada	205	54	Panama	22	5
United States of America	197	54	Saint Vincent	20	0
Australia	182	51	Grenadine	17	—
Puerto Rico	176	23	Santa Lucia	17	0
Scotland	166	60	Iran	16	4
Uruguay	159	—	Belize	13	—
New Zealand	157	50	Kuwait	12	5
El Salvador	148	61	Bahamas	10	—
Singapore	147	107	Guatemala	9	1
Netherlands	146	81	Philippines	5	4
Korea	139	49	Syria	2	—
Hong Kong	137	107	Papua New Guinea	1	2
Portugal	136	51	Egypt	0	0
Northern Ireland	131	39	Malta	*	6
England and Wales	121	57	Dem. Rep. Germany	*	—
			Cuba	*	—

Notes:
Figures taken from WHO Statistics Annual (1987), latest year of reporting.
*No figures reported in WHO Statistics Annual 1987.

Notable exceptions to the reporting states are the People's Republic of China, the USSR, and most African nations. Secondly, the validity of the figures reported is questionable for a number of reasons which will be discussed in the concluding section of this chapter.

Of particular note is that in every country the rate of suicide for males is higher, and most of the time considerably higher, than for females. Barraclough (1988), in his anaysis of WHO annual statistics over the period 1973–85, found equal or higher rates for

15–24-year-old women in four Asian countries (i.e. Thailand, Hong Kong, Philippines, and Singapore). As will be shown later in this chapter, this reversal of the classic sex distribution in suicide appears to be limited to the 15–24-year-old age group.

International changes in suicide rates 1960–80/6

For a number of the industrialised countries in the Western hemisphere, an increase in suicide rates has been reported over the last decades (Diekstra, 1985). Table 2 illustrates how common this trend is at a global level. For the sixty-two countries which reported to WHO both in 1960 and at least in one of the years 1980–6 the respective suicide rates are presented.

TABLE 2a: Suicide rates (per 100 000 of population in sixty-two countries, 1960[a]

Country	*Rate*	*Country*	*Rate*
1. Fed. Rep. Germany	37	32. Chile	7.5
2. Hungary	25	33. Argentina	7.4
3. Austria	23.1	34. Martinique	6.8
4. Czechoslovakia	22.3	35. Netherlands	6.6
5. Japan	21.6	36. Suriname	6.5
6. Finland	20.5	37. Norway	6.4
7. Denmark	20.3	38. Venezuela	6.1
8. Switzerland	29.2	39. Italy	6.1
9. Dem. Rep. Germany	28.6	40. Spain	5.5
10. Sweden	17.4	41. Panama	4.1
11. France	15.8	42. N. Ireland	4.4
12. Belgium	14.6	43. Greece	4.3
13. Yugoslvia	13.9	44. Guadeloupe	3.9
14. Luxembourg	13.4	45. Thailand	3.5
15. Uruguay	12.7	46. Mauritius	3.5
16. El Salvador	12.1	47. Trinidad & Tabago	3.2
17. England & Wales	11.2	48. Ireland	3.0
18. Hong Kong	11.1	49. Colombia	2.7
19. Cuba	11.1	50. Guatemala	2.7
20. United States of America	10.6	51. Costa Rica	2.5
21. Australia	10.6	52. Jamaica	2.0
22. Iceland	10.6	53. Mexico	1.9
23. Puerto Rico	10.3	54. Antigua & Barbuda	1.8
24. Sri Lanka	9.9	55. Peru	1.5
25. New Zealand	9.7	56. Malta	0.9
26. Bulgaria	8.7	57. Ecuador	0.8
27. Portugal	8.7	58. Dominican Republic	0.8
28. Singapore	8.6	59. Philippines	0.7
29. Poland	8.0	60. Nicaragua	0.4
30. Scotland	7.9	61. Egypt	0.1
31. Canada	7.6	62. Papua New Guinea	0.1

Note:
[a]WHO Data bank latest year of reporting as per 1 July 1988.

TABLE 2b: Suicide rates (per 100 000 of population) in sixty-two countries, 1980–6[a]

Country	*Rate*	*Country*	*Rate*
1. Hungary	45.3	32. Uruguay	9.6
2. Fed. Rep. Germany	43.1	33. Northern Ireland	9.3
3. Sri Lanka	29	34. Portugal	9.2
4. Austria	28.3	35. England & Wales	8.9
5. Denmark	27.8	36. Trinidad & Tobago	8.6
6. Finland	26.6	37. Guadeloupe	7.9
7. Belgium	23.8	38. Ireland	7.8
8. Switzerland	22.8	39. Italy	7.6
9. France	22.7	40. Thailand	6.6
10. Suriname	21.6	41. Argentina	6.3
11. Japan	21.2	42. Chile	6.2
12. Dem. Rep. Germany	19.0	43. Spain	4.9
13. Czechoslovakia	18.9	44. Venezuela	4.8
14. Sweden	18.5	45. Costa Rica	4.5
15. Cuba	17.7	46. Ecuador	4.3
16. Bulgaria	16.3	47. Greece	4.1
17. Yugoslavia	16.1	48. Martinique	3.7
18. Norway	14.1	49. Colombia	2.9
19. Luxenbourg	13.9	50. Mauritius	2.8
20. Iceland	13.3	51. Dominican Republic	2.4
21. Poland	13.0	52. Mexico	1.6
22. Canada	12.9	53. Panama	1.4
23. Singapore	12.7	54. Peru	1.4
24. United States of America	12.3	55. Philippines	0.5
25. Hong Kong	12.2	56. Guatemala	0.5
26. Australia	11.6	57. Malta	0.3
27. Scotland	11.6	58. Nicaragua	0.2
28. Netherlands	11.0	59. Papua New Guinea	0.2
29. El Salvador	10.8	60. Jamaica	0.1
30. New Zealand	10.3	61. Egypt	0.1
31. Puerto Rico	9.8	62. Antigua & Barbuda	—

Note:
[a]WHO Data bank latest year of reporting as per 1 July 1988.

A comparison of the rates for 1960 and 1985 indicates that about twenty-five years ago the rank order of the countries was somewhat, but not very much, different from today's ranking. This is true in spite of the often substantial changes in suicide rates (see Table 3). It appears that more countries (forty-two) have witnessed an increase than a decrease (twenty) in suicide rates over the past twenty to twenty-five years. The average percentage change is about 37 per cent with a range of 66 per cent to 437 per cent. The logical conclusion to draw from this data is that suicide mortality on a global level has apparently increased over the last quarter of a century. However, closer inspection of Table 3 in conjunction with Tables 2a and 2b shows a remarkable pattern.

Relatively large increases are observed in most countries in

TABLE 3: Per cent change in mortality by suicide in sixty-two countries between 1960 and 1986

Country	*Rate*	*Country*	*Rate*
1. Hungary	81	32. Uruguay	−24
2. Fed. Rep. Germany	2	33. Northern Ireland	111
3. Sri Lanka	193	34. Portugal	6
4. Austria	25.5	35. England & Wales	21
5. Denmark	37	36. Trinidad & Tobago	169
6. Finland	30	37. Guadeloupe	102
7. Belgium	63	38. Ireland	160
8. Switzerland	19	39. Italy	25
9. France	44	40. Thailand	89
10. Suriname	232	41. Argentina	−15
11. Japan	−2	42. Chile	−17
12. Dem. Rep. Germany	2	43. Spain	−11
13. Czechoslovakia	−15	44. Venezuela	−21
14. Sweden	6	45. Costa Rica	80
15. Cuba	59	46. Ecuador	437
16. Bulgaria	87	47. Greece	−5
17. Yugoslavia	16	48. Martinique	−46
18. Norway	120	49. Colombia	7
19. Luxembourg	4	50. Mauritius	−20
20. Iceland	25	51. Dominican Republic	200
21. Poland	62	52. Mexico	−16
22. Canada	70	53. Panama	−66
23. Singapore	48	54. Peru	−7
24. United States of America	16	55. Philippines	−29
25. Hong Kong	1	56. Guatemala	−82
26. Australia	9	57. Malta	−67
27. Scotland	41	58. Nicaragua	−50
28. Netherlands	67	59. Papua New Guinea	100
29. El Salvador	−15	60. Jamaica	−50
30. New Zealand	6	61. Egypt	0
31. Peurto Rico	−6	62. Antigua & Barbuda	—

North-west and Central Europe. Countries populated in the majority by European descent show a similar trend, though generally less sizeable. Striking is the fact that the Latin countries, both around the Mediterranean as well as on the American continent, witness decreasing suicide rates. For the Asian countries the picture is mixed with relatively large increases for South-East Asia (Sri Lanka, Thailand, and Singapore) and no changes or decreases for the Far East (Hong Kong, Japan, and the Philippines).

Such a strikingly consistent geographic distribution of changes in suicide rates in the world suggests that they are probably not simply a reflection of changes in classification procedures but rather a consequence of socio-cultural developments, the nature of which remains obscure.

The relationship of age and sex with suicide rates

As has been mentioned earlier in this chapter, the total suicide rates for males are higher than for females in every country reported in the *World Health Statistics Annual*, 1987. This picture remains the same if one looks at different age groups. Tables 4(a, b) show the rates for a selected number of countries (nineteen) for three different age groups (15–29, 30–59, 60 and over) for males and females separately for 1970, and again for the latest year of reporting (1986 or 1986).

It appears that in only one of the fifty-seven possible comparisons, the female suicide rate exceeds the rate for males (Singapore, 1970, age group 15–29).[4] For many of the countries the gender gap seems to be widening over the period 1970 to 1985–6. In the age range 15–29 the rates for males have gone up in sixteen countries, with only two (Czechoslovakia and Venezuela) showing a decrease and one (Hungary) no change. For females in this age group, seven countries show decreasing rates. The differences in trends between the sexes are less striking for the other two age groups, although here the number of countries as well as the magnitude of the increase is greater for males.

Generally speaking, for both sexes the increase in suicide rates over the period (1970–1985/6) is strongest for the 15–29 year olds, although there are some exceptions to this rule that are noteworthy. For example, in Japan the total suicide rate shows a decline that is reflected in all age and sex subgroups with the exception of males between 30–59 years of age. Their rate has almost doubled in a relatively short period of about fifteen years. Something similar, although at a less dramatic level, is found for Hungarian males, who have a stable rate for the age group 15–29 and a considerable increase in the 30–59 year olds. For females this same pattern is found in Singapore.

The data in Tables 4(a, b) confirm the general observation that suicide rates increase with advancing age. The countries where this regularity is violated include two Latin American countries, Venezuela and Mexico, where both in 1970 and 1985, young females aged 15–29 have the highest rates. Remarkable also is the fact that in 1986, males aged 15–29 in Australia and New Zealand have higher rates than males aged 30–59. This is a consequence of a strong increase in the suicide rate for the first and a decrease in the latter age group. In other countries, including Canada, the United States of America, and Ireland, a somewhat similar de-

TABLE 4a: Suicide in females 1970 and 1985–6

Country	1970 15–29	1970 30–59	1970 60+	1985–6 15–29	1985–6 30–59	1985–6 60+
1. Australia	6.2	12.4	12.3	5.3	6.9	8.4
2. Belgium	3.4	15.1	25.7	6.5	21.3	26.2
3. Bulgaria	5.0	8.5	27.7	5.7	8.0	31.3
4. Canada	5.9	10.3	6.9	4.6	8.3	6.3
5. Czechoslovakia	11.5	15.4	35.5	4.8	10.3	27.0
6. Denmark	6.4	25.4	23.3	9.9	30.4	29.5
7. England & Wales	2.9	8.9	11.9	10.5	7.6	17.7
8. France	5.4	10.3	18.2	6.3	16.2	26.2
9. W. Germany	8.1	20.7	26.6	6.6	12.6	23.1
10. Hungary	9.6	20.8	59.3	11.3	29.7	65.7
11. Ireland	0.3	1.1	1.1	1.2	6.3	5.1
12. Japan	12.8	13.4	53.0	9.5	10.3	45.5
13. Mexico	1.0	0.7	0.3	1.4	0.9	0.7
14. Netherlands	3.3	9.3	15.3	5.4	11.9	12.5
15. New Zealand	4.1	10.9	14.9	6.0	7.0	6.1
16. Scotland	2.5	11.2	6.1	3.4	7.0	10.4
17. Singapore	10.9	7.9	56.3	8.0	12.7	69.4
18. USA	6.0	11.7	8.3	4.7	7.6	6.5
19. Venezuela	9.0	4.1	5.2	10.9	2.7	2.7

WHO databank.

TABLE 4b: Suicide in males 1970 and 1985–6

Country	1970 15–29	1970 30–59	1970 60+	1985–6 15–29	1985–6 30–59	1985–6 60+
1. Australia	15.3	29.1	33.2	26.1	22.3	28.6
2. Belgium	8.8	27.0	76.0	22.7	38.6	85.8
3. Bulgaria	9.8	16.2	82.5	14.0	22.8	102.5
4. Canada	17.1	27.1	23.9	25.6	26.2	28.2
5. Czechoslovakia	32.5	52.3	87.9	18.1	43.4	79.7
6. Denmark	15.3	44.7	50.0	24.3	47.1	72.5
7. England & Wales	6.7	13.0	21.4	10.5	16.7	19.9
8. France	11.3	32.2	68.5	22.7	41.5	93.7
9. W. Germany	22.8	39.5	67.7	19.7	32.3	59.2
10. Hungary	33.2	70.6	131.3	33.5	98.3	156.9
11. Ireland	2.8	5.0	4.2	15.9	15.9	16.1
12. Japan	16.5	20.8	70.2	18.4	40.3	64.7
13. Mexico	3.1	3.4	5.8	4.3	4.1	9.6
14. Netherlands	6.0	14.1	35.1	10.0	17.7	37.7
15. New Zealand	11.1	21.2	26.8	19.6	18.5	33.1
16. Scotland	6.7	14.9	20.8	15.8	23.4	21.1
17. Singapore	10.4	20.3	98.4	12.7	18.1	99.4
18. USA	16.2	25.4	39.3	22.6	23.6	43.4
19. Venezuela	14.6	17.4	19.1	10.9	13.4	23.4

WHO databank.

velopment can be observed in that the rates of males 15–29 are approximately the same as the rates for 30–59 year olds. For females the same trend can be observed in England and Wales, and Australia and New Zealand. It is of interest to note that all these countries are predominantly Anglo-Saxon. This suggests that there may be common factors operating in the Anglo-Saxon part of the world that might be contributory to the phenomenon.

One country, Czechoslovakia, particularly stands out because it is the only country that shows declining suicide rates over the period 1970–85 for all age and sex groups. One explanation for this might be that in 1968 this country had witnessed the invasion and occupation by the armies of the Warsaw Pact countries, which evoked desperate reactions, especially by young people (e.g. the self-burning by Jan Palach at the Wenceslas Square in 1968, shortly after the invasion). By 1985 there was a new generation of adolescents and young adults who had not experienced the aftermath of this traumatic event. The fact that the drop in suicide rate is the greatest among the 15–29 year olds appears to lend some support to this hypothesis.

The importance of suicide as a cause of death

Tables 5(a, b) show a breakdown in three age groups of the percentage of all deaths caused by suicide for a selected number of countries. The age groups have been chosen to represent the two groups with the highest and the one group with the lowest percen-

TABLE 5a: Suicide in males as a percentage of all death causes in that age

Country	*Age*			
	15–24	*25–34*	*65–74*	*all ages*
Australia	17.7	20.3	0.5	2.2
Bulgaria	10.8	9.6	1.1	1.7
Czechoslovakia	13.0	20.0	1.0	2.3
Canada	20.7	20.6	0.8	2.6
Denmark	18.6	28.2	1.4	2.9
England & Wales	10.9	18.1	0.4	1.0
France	13.9	21.7	1.7	3.1
Hungary	18.8	27.8	2.0	4.4
Ireland	9.0	14.3	0.4	0.9
Japan	19.5	29.6	1.6	4.1
Netherlands	15.2	21.5	0.7	1.6
New Zealand	12.8	14.4	0.9	1.8
Scotland	16.6	17.4	0.5	1.3
Singapore	12.6	13.6	1.2	2.6
USA	14.5	14.3	0.9	2.1

WHO databank.

TABLE 5b: Suicide in females as a percentage of all causes of death

Country	*Age*			
	15–24	*25–34*	*65–74*	*all ages*
Australia	10.3	8.5	0.1	0.7
Bulgaria	9.9	7.9	0.8	0.9
Czechoslovakia	10.4	13.5	0.7	0.8
Canada	9.6	12.5	0.4	0.9
Denmark	23.3	25.0	1.5	1.9
England & Wales	6.2	9.5	0.5	0.5
France	10.1	16.2	1.7	1.4
Hungary	18.8	18.6	1.6	2.0
Ireland	8.5	7.0	0.2	0.5
Japan	28.0	24.9	2.3	2.7
Netherlands	11.2	10.5	0.9	1.0
New Zealand	9.0	7.3	0.4	0.6
Scotland	9.4	11.1	0.5	0.5
Singapore	15.0	17.6	0.6	2.5
USA	8.6	8.9	0.3	0.7

WHO databank.

tage. Two facts emerge very clearly. First of all, the 25–34-year-old age group has the highest relative mortality risk from suicide. In some countries, such as Japan and Denmark, approximately one in every three males and one out of every four females who die in that age group does so by suicide. Secondly, two Asian countries, Singapore and Japan, are the only countries in the world in which the relative mortality by suicide is higher for females than for males among 15–24 year olds. In Singapore this is also true for the 25–34 age group. This distinct difference from other countries in the world, especially Europe and North America, might well reflect cultural differences regarding the position of women in these societies (Barraclough, 1988; Headley, 1983).

The complexity of cause and cure

One obvious conclusion from this analysis of international suicide rates is that there is much unexplained variation between countries in the incidence of suicide. A second conclusion is that as far as trends are concerned, many countries show a considerable to very strong increase in the frequency of suicide in the 15–29-year-age group over the past two decades. This tendency is especially strong in European states, but is also clearly present in North America, Asia, Oceania, and in certain Latin American countries. It is stronger for males than females.

TABLE 6: Multiple causes of suicidal behaviour

Cause	*Example*
Physiological predisposition	Male gender (suicide), genetic/biological disorders, high emotional/high inhibition temperament type, physical illness
Cultural context	Societal norms, traditions encouraging/restraining suicidal behaviour
Socio-economic context	Economic deprivation, unemployment, breakdown of social infrastructure
Immediate interpersonal environment	Overcrowding, urban stress
Personal characteristics	Psychiatric or personality disorders, cognitive constriction, addictive behaviour
Disinhibitors	Alcohol, drugs, current suicidal models
Presence of means	Guns, drugs, other means
Presence of potential rescuer	Spouse, child, parent, other

Despite numerous efforts to explain international differences in suicide rates and trends to date, there exists no generally accepted explanatory theory—nor even a small selected group of competitive theories supported by different groups of researchers. What does clearly emerge from the literature is that suicides, and for that matter, parasuicides, are highly complex phenomena both geno- and phenotypically. The search for one responsible age, a 'suicidococcus', has proved to be unfruitful. Every act of suicidal behaviour has multiple causes, that is, it grows from an array of societal and individual factors.

In broad outline, Table 6 presents a possible way of highlighting the complexity of causation of suicidal behaviour, indicating the necessity of parallel complexity of solution. The call for complexity of solution has been heard before in a number of other areas, such as aggression reduction, from community psychologists, ecological psychologists, environmental designers, systems analysts, and health policy-makers in international organisations such as the WHO. It has, however, relatively seldom been heard in the area of suicidology until now, presumably because of the fact that most of the work with regard to intervention and prevention of suicidal behaviour has mainly remained within the realm of clinical settings. Although in recent years some authors have proposed approaching the problem of the prevention of suicidal behaviour from a broader community perspective (Diekstra and Hawton, 1987), most of the interventions are prevention activities which have usually taken the form of rather isolated projects, such as school curricula for suicide education. Apart from the danger that such activities might be counter-productive because they might not only provide information on suicidal behaviour but also provide models for that behaviour, they also have the disadvantage of not being directed towards those population groups which carry the highest risk for suicidal behaviour, especially for completed suicide. Besides, they might be applicable and useful in certain, mainly developed, countries, while at the same time not being applicable in other countries or parts of countries, especially in the developing world. The ability to generalise such activities may be further limited by the fact that cultures differ widely with regard to their attitudes towards suicidal behaviour and, therefore, to the acceptability of programmes that speak openly and frankly about it. From an international and a WHO point of view, therefore, the view is that to have even modest chance of enduring success of preventing self-destructive behaviour, programmes designed to reduce that behaviour must be oriented not only to the level of the individual but also the levels of the family, school, work-place, and other larger scale organisations, as well as the larger community context. Furthermore, an optimal complex prevention programme designed to reduce suicide rates ought to seek to do so via a variety of modes or channels. It may well be that one of the reasons why intervention and prevention programmes in a number of countries have not withstood empirical tests of their efficacy is that they have not been based on the 'complex cause-complex cure' approach (WHO, 1982). Simply put, complex problems require complex solutions.

The growing awareness of that effect has recently led in a few countries (Canada, United States of America and the Netherlands) to the establishment of national task forces on suicide, which have been charged with the task of devising comprehensive national programmes for the prevention of suicidal behaviour. The recommendations of these task forces, as far as they have published in preliminary or final form (Syer-Solursh, 1986; US Task Force Report, 1988; Simmons, 1987; Diekstra, 1986), are generally in line with the recommendations made by the World Health Organization (WHO, 1982). It is for this reason that in the remainder of this chapter the four main categories of recommendations to emerge from these national and international strategies will be briefly described.

Towards a comprehensive strategy for the prevention of suicidal behaviour

Both from an international as well as a national or country perspective prevention of suicidal behaviour depends on the degree to which the following four conditions are met:

(*1*) the assembly of scientifically sound information on the causation of suicidal behaviour, on efficacy of intervention and prevention schemes, and on effective methodologies for implementing such schemes in a variety of cultural and socio-economical situations;

(*2*) the improvement of services dealing with suicidal persons or persons at high risk for suicidal behaviour;

(*3*) the effective provision of information and training to relevant organisations and the general public; and

(*4*) the provision of special services to high-risk groups.

Each of these conditions will now be described in more detail.

Research

There is an urgent need for more and better information concerning the causes of suicidal behaviour, the factors causing international differences in rates, risk factors involved, and methods of preventing suicidal behaviour. Compared with other health problems, the amount of knowledge available in this field is extremely limited. The necessary information, if effective intervention and prevention programmes are to be set up, must be selected by means of carefully designed and implemented national and international research programmes. Essential components of such a programme should be as follows.

(*1*) The collection at national and international level of valid and up-to-date data concerning the incidence of suicide and suicide attempts and the characteristics of individuals who make suicide attempts, whether with a fatal or non-fatal outcome, should be established. For this it is necessary that:

> (*a*) the classification/certification of suicidal behaviour be improved through the international adoption of uniform definitions and operational criteria for suicide and suicide attempts, preferably in systems like the International Classification of Diseases (WHO, 1978);

(*b*) measures be taken to ensure that the authorities/persons whose responsibility it is to establish suicide as the cause of death do in fact apply the criteria referred to under (*a*);
(*c*) data collection at the national and international level be developed in such a way that the information can be used for analytical–epidemiological studies of the characteristics of high-risk groups and the changes in those characteristics which take place over time;
(*d*) data collection be done in such a way that the effects of local and regional prevention or intervention programmes can be tested;
(*e*) general hospitals and other medical and social services which treat suicide attempts be encouraged to maintain records of these cases, which can be regularly reviewed by a regional or local body.

(*2*) There should be funding of a carefully designed multidisciplinary international research programme in which a range of relevant risk factors for suicidal behaviour are investigated. The programme must be planned and directed in such a way that existing research projects and available knowledge are made use of and to provide the information necessary for effective prevention or intervention programmes. It should also study, among other things, the interaction between multiple risk factors, such as emotional disturbance and alcohol and drug abuse, as well as the question of whether there is a causal relationship between biological, environmental, and cultural factors and suicidal behaviour.

(*3*) There should be well-planned research studies using control groups which examine methods for treating suicide attempters and of prevention programmes for high-risk groups (e.g. relatives and close friends of people who have committed suicide).

(*4*) There should also be carefully planned studies into the most effective and safe way of informing the public about suicide and into the positive and negative effects the media can produce in this context.

Improving services

It is of great importance that available services designed to help people with a high risk of suicidal behaviour be expanded and improved. This should occur within the public mental health system, the welfare and social services, *and* the judicial/law enforcement agencies. Pending the results of research into the effectiveness of methods of prevention and intervention, improvements can be made in a number of areas such as the following.

(*1*) Increased competence of professionals in the health and mental health system who identify and treat suicidal and depressed persons must be increased. This means that the training for physicians, psychiatrists, clinical and health psychologists, psychotherapists, social workers, and general and social/psychiatric nurses must include the following obligatory components:

(*a*) information on the epidemiology of suicide and attempted suicide and acute and chronic risk factors of suicidal behaviour;

(*b*) information on, and training in, the skills necessary to identify people with a high risk of suicidal behaviour;

(*c*) training in interview techniques, treatment and after-care of suicidal people, relatives of people who have committed suicide, and the families of friends of people who have made a suicide attempt;

(*d*) training in the appropriate referral of suicidal people to (other) health care workers.

(*2*) Models/scenarios should be developed to assist institutions and staff within the health and mental health system to give more specific and better co-ordinated assistance/after-care to suicidal people and their relatives.

One way to achieve this goal is to make community mental (health) systems on the primary health care level responsible for the co-ordination of care/treatment of suicidal persons and for developing models which will ensure that the following tasks are fulfilled:

(*a*) the provision of direct and specific assistance and intervention in crisis situations;

(*b*) the making of thorough assessments of suicide risk and appropriate plans for treatment;

(*c*) the referral and transfer of suicidal people to other services and the provision of appropriate help and after-care by various agencies;

(*d*) the provision of mental health consultations for dealing with suicidal persons and their relatives to health care workers;

(*e*) the maintenance of records to monitor the extent of the problem and to evaluate the care provided.

The implications of the above recommendations are that the primary health care level will assume a co-ordinating role in assuring that appropriate expertise and sufficient access to services are available within each community. Primary health care workers/agencies will have to establish contact with other relevant services available in the community (police, general practitioners, emergency telephone services, social health services, ambulance services, etc.) and ensure collaboration with in-patient health care institutions (general hospitals, psychiatric units in general hospitals, general psychiatric hospital, university psychiatric clinics). Every effort must be made to ensure that the designated agency's address and telephone number in a community becomes so well known and so accessible that it can operate as the central point from which immediate assistance in case of emergencies can be obtained.

Measures should also be taken to ensure the following.

(*1*) In every hospital providing medical (emergency) treatment for attempted suicides, a formal policy should be established with regard to psychiatric assessment, treatment, and referral of suicide attempters and their relatives.

(*2*) The help given to suicide attempters in hospitals should be organized to incorporate clinical psychiatric and psychological knowledge and skills and expertise in crisis intervention.

(*3*) Facilities should be established for prolonged observation of suicidal persons in hospitals, even when medical treatment has ended.

(*4*) Formal arrangements should be made between the primary health care facilities and in-patient psychiatric institutions for the referral and after-care of suicide attempters and their relatives;

(*5*) In order to improve further the care provided to suicide attempters in general psychiatric hospitals:

(*a*) research should be carried out into the short-term and long-term factors which have contributed to the rise in the suicide rate in such hospitals;

(*b*) greater emphasis should be placed on training people to work with suicidal patients in psychiatric hospitals. More attention should be devoted to health care workers' own attitudes towards suicide. In this regard, research into effective treatment methods for patients who repeatedly attempt suicide is of great importance.

(*c*) Training and information regarding the problem of suicide.

The provision of appropriate information and training to relevant organisations/groups and the general public is essential if the suicide rate is to be reduced substantially and to mitigate effects on survivors. The following points are worthy of particular consideration:

(*1*) Curricula of primary and secondary school teachers, counsellors, and career teachers should include information and training on assessing severe depression and the risk of suicide and appropriate referral of suicidal pupils. The same holds true for the curricula of workers dealing with out-of-schoolers or school dropouts. Relevant curricula models must include:

(*a*) information concerning the acute and chronic risk factors associated with suicidal behaviour;

(*b*) information on the characteristic symptoms of depression and other psychological disturbances as they may be manifested within the school context;

(*c*) information on criteria and methods for referral of students who are clearly at risk and identification of referral institutions;

(*d*) training in interpersonal and communication skills necessary to approach and establish an understanding relationship with such pupils; and

(*e*) information on how linkages between mental health services and the schools can best deal with, and respond to, suicide or attempted suicide by pupils.

(*2*) With regard to the role of the police, the following recommendations are made:

(*a*) senior police officials should ensure that in the event of a suicide, or an attempted suicide, police duties be carried out, wherever possible, by officers who have the necessary skills and appropriate attitudes;

(*b*) policies and guidelines should be established, based upon police experience, which can be followed in cases of suicide and attempted suicide—these might include the wearing of civilian clothes, providing support to surviving relatives until other helpers arrive, and contacting the family physician;

(*c*) arrangements must be made to ensure that items seized at the time of a suicide (such as suicide notes, diaries, and other evidence of a personal nature) are returned to the family as soon as investigations have been completed.

(*3*) In order to assess the role of emergency telephone services and their potential in suicide prevention, research should be undertaken:

(*a*) to investigate how the role of emergency telephone services can be optimally used to prevent suicide. The focus should be on such aspects as the training of volunteer workers, the telephone services' relationship with agencies providing assistance, and on the linkage to mental health professionals;

(*b*) to study the long-term follow-up of the suicidal persons who have contacted emergency telephone services. The information obtained should help to clarify the role of telephone services to determine whether they require more governmental support than is currently the case.

(*4*) With regard to the general public, it is indicated that efforts are needed to increase the awareness of the symptoms of depression and other warnings of suicide. In addition, more publicity should be given to organisations which can offer confidential and professional advice and/or assistance to suicidal persons and their families.

(*5*) The role of the media with regard to the above-mentioned points (*1–4*) can be very significant but may also provoke or encourage suicidal behaviour. It is recommended that, in the interests of suicide prevention, the media should exercise great prudence and restraint in news items concerning suicide and in publishing articles or broadcasting programmes concerning cases of suicidal behaviour. It should be the rule that such material and the method of presentation are discussed with experts in suicidal behaviour and prevention before it is made public.

Special groups

For certain special groups it is suggested that the following provisions be made.

(*1*) Provisions for identifying and preventing suicidal behaviour among adolescents should be clearly organised and should take the form of:

(*a*) in the case of school-attending adolescents, collaboration between schools and the primary mental health services within each community; where possible parents should be involved. Furthermore, arranging for a psychiatrist or psychologist to consult at the school on certain days with pupils who have psychological problems would be advisable; and

(*b*) in the case of youngsters not attending school special community outreach activities should be established.

(*2*) Care of the potentially suicidal elderly should include an active outreach policy directed at elderly people living alone and, in particular, those who have recently experienced the death of their partner. These programmes must be set up as part of primary health care services. Efforts must be made to make regular checks on the physical condition of the widow or widower (which can often deteriorate rapidly after the death of the partner) and to encourage socialisation of the person. Such an approach is of particular importance with childless elderly couples and should be continued for at least a year after the death of the partner. The various agencies involved must (under the co-ordination of primary health care agencies) establish clear policies at regional levels regarding such activities.

It is further recommended that regional geriatric services provide better information about depressive disorders and their treatment to health care professionals and to the elderly.

(*3*) More research is needed on suicidal behaviour in correctional institutions and prisons, particularly into methods of preventing such behaviour. Better training of prison staff to identify and intervene with suicidal inmates is also needed.

(*4*) It is recommended that health care professionals who care for the chronically ill should be trained to identify and to discuss suicidal thoughts and plans with patients, to assess the risk of suicidal behaviour, to evaluate the degree to which suicidal wishes are related to acceptance of illness or disability and the extent to which an acceptable quality of life, given the disability, is possible. They must also be trained in counselling such patients, or where this is not part of their job, in referring them appropriately.

(*5*) Agencies and individuals involved in treating alcoholics and substance abusers should be alert to the risk of suicide among their patients/clients and should be trained to identify and deal with an increased risk of suicidal behaviour. To enhance suicide prevention efforts, it is important that national measures be taken to combate alcohol and drug abuse.

(*6*) Relatives of people who have committed suicide should be considered at high risk for suicide and, therefore, an important target group for preventive measures. Given that they do not often ask for help themselves, an active approach must be used to contact and assist them. It is an important responsibility of the primary mental health services to get in touch with relatives of people who have committed suicide as soon as possible after the event to offer help and to repeat this offer in subsequent contacts. These supporting interventions should continue for at least a year after the suicide.

Assistance should include both individual help and counselling for the surviving family members as a group. Primary health care agencies should organise grief work groups for survivors of those who have committed suicide to facilitate their working through their bereavement and grief.

Additionally, information (e.g. brochures) should be immediately made available to survivors describing in simple terms the process of coming to terms with complex feelings of grief, loss and guilt, social consequences and ways of dealing with them, as well as ways of seeking help from others. An assessement of community organisation provisions for dealing with suicidal people should be made. Where services are immediate it is recommended that the federal or state governments request these organisations to make such provisions.

Conclusions

Suicide is an international problem, touching virtually every country in the world. Suicide and attempted suicide can be prevented, but the development and evaluation of effective large-scale prevention programmes is still in its infancy. The organisational structures required for well-co-ordinated programmes of research and practice in the area of suicide prevention are yet to be built. Training of health care professionals and other relevant groups in the assessment and management of suicide risk is still lacking. These inadequacies in current programmes across the world have promoted the establishment of national Task Forces on Suicide Prevention in the United States of America, Canada, and the Netherlands, as well as a WHO strategy on suicide prevention. These groups have formulated comprehensive strategies for the prevention of suicide. The main components of these strategies are: (*a*) the design and implementation of national research programmes; (*b*) the improvement of services; (*c*) the provision of information and training on suicide prevention to relevant professional groups, organisations, and the general public; and (*d*) the formulation of strategies and techniques to deal with special risk groups.

Notes

1. Because national statistics on parasuicide are not available,

this chapter discusses only international differences and trends in suicide.

2. For reasons of convenience the term country or state in this chapter means any territory with mortality statistics reported to WHO Headquarters, Geneva.
3. Although the data for the Falklands are suspect, there is presently no evidence that the figure is due to misreporting or recording error.
4. In contrast with Barraclough's findings (1988), Thailand, Hong Kong, and the Philippines do not appear in this list, which is due to the fact that he used the 15–24 years age range.

References

Barraclough, B. (1988). 'International Variation in the Suicide Rate of 15–24-year-olds', *Soc Psychiat*, 23, 75–84.

Diekstra, R.F.W. (1982). 'Epidemilogy of Attempted Suicide in the EEC', in J. Wilmott, and J. Mendlewicz (eds.), *New Trends in Suicide Prevention*, Basel: Bibliotheca Psychiatrica, Karger, 1–16.

—— (1985). 'Suicide and Suicide Attempts in the European Economic Community: An Analysis of Trends with Special Emphasis on Trends among the Young', *Suicd Lifethr B*, 15, 402–21.

—— *et al.* (1986). *Rapport inzake suicide* (*Report on Suicide*), December, The Hague: Health Council of the Netherlands.

Simmons, K. (1987). Task Force to Make Recommendations for Adolescents in Terms of Suicide Risk', *Jauna*, 257, 3330–2.

Syer-Solursh, D., personal communications (1986). US Department of Health and Human Services.

WHO (1978). *International Classification of Diseases* (ICD-9), Geneva: World Health Organization.

WHO (1982). Changing Patterns in Suicide Behaviour', *WHO/EURO Reports and Studies*, 74, Copenhagen.

WHO (1987). *World Health Statistics Annual*, Geneva: World Health Organization.

WHO (1988). *Correlates of Youth Suicide*, Technical Document, Geneva: World Health Organization, Division of Mental Health.

The sociology of suicide in Hungary

P. HARMAT

Hungary's suicide rate has been high ever since the early nineteenth century, and since 1968 the highest in the world. In the second half of the 1940s the suicide rate was 23.7 per 100 000 population on the five-year average. This was a quite low figure in this century.

In the early 1950s, when Hungary was under a harsh Stalinist dictatorship, the suicide rate dropped to 21.5, which was the lowest five-year average in the country in this century. In the second half of the 1950s, the rate grew to 23 per 100 000 and in the first half of the 1960s to over 27. These latter years are known in Hungary as the years of consolidation, rising living standards and an easing of domestic tensions. Notwithstanding this, in 1967 the suicide rate was above 30 per 100 000 and by 1968 Hungary topped the world statistics with a rate of 33.7. Within a century, Hungary moved from fifteenth to first place in the world's suicide rate statistics. And it seems that rather than being due to certain methodological peculiarities, this eminence corresponds to the facts (Sainsbury and Barraclough, 1968).

The upward trend did not stop in 1968. In the 1980s, the rate fluctuated between 44.4 and 45.9. Halbwachs had already suggested in 1930 that there must be an end somewhere to the growth in suicide rate, and it appears that this finally came about in Hungary after 1980. Between 1968 and 1980 in only two years, 1973 and 1975, were there fewer suicides (and in 1973 the drop was minimal, with only seven suicides less); since 1980 there have been three years showing a decline, namely, 1982, 1984, and 1985. The 1986 rate also failed to reach the 1983 record figure of 45.9. In other words, the signs indicate that in the first half of the 1980s the Hungarian suicide rate has levelled off, albeit at a very high rate (Andorka *et al.* 1986).

The high suicide rate has given rise to much public concern. There are serious debates concerning the reasons behind this phenomenon. Often in the course of the past century, the issue of the suicide rate has become part of ongoing social criticism and political controversies, compared with which the intensity of scientific investigation leaves much to be desired.

What are the sociological and epidemiological details of Hungary's suicide rate? The rate of suicide among the elderly, that is, those over 65 years of age, is several times that of the 15–24 age category. In 1984, in the case of men it was five times as high and in that of women 9.5 times as high. The ageing of the population—due to the declining birth rate—is only partly (approximately a third) responsible for the rising suicide rate of the past several decades.

Recent research has shown an unusually high rate among those who were 20–24 years old at the time of the Second World War (Szigeti, 1986). Members of this group were born in the late 1910s and early 1920s, and since 1945 have committed suicide at a disproportionately high rate.

At the same time, the youth suicide rate is also high in Hungary. In 1984, Hungary ranked second behind in Austria in terms of the 15–24 age group, surpassing the high Czechoslovak, West German, Danish, and Swedish rates.

For many years, Budapest had a higher suicide rate than rural Hungary, and the capital was considered a suicide centre (Andorka, Cseh-Szombathy and Vavró, 1968). Then a gradual shift set in, to the point at which the difference first disappeared, then by 1979 tipped towards the rural regions. In 1960, the nation's suicide rate in terms of location showed a declining tendency in the following order: Budapest, county seats, district townships, villages. By 1984, this was: villages, Budapest and county seats (no difference in rates), small towns. In Budapest, the suicide rate is especially high in the decaying inner city.

The highest suicide rate is found in south-eastern Hungary, in regions to the east of the River Tisza and between the Tisza and the Danube. The next highest are regions in northern Hungary and in Transdanubia (Andorka, Cseh-Szombathy and Vavró, 1968; Cseh-Szombathy, 1963; Jobb, 1973). For example, in 1984 in Bács-Kiskún County, which tops the list, the rate was 73.8, while in Vas

County, at the bottom of the list, it was 20.2 per 100 000 population. This regional discrepancy is not due to differences in the age groups of the respective counties but to local traditions of suicide, the preponderance of different religious denominations, the system of scattered farmsteads, the absence or presence of closed peasant communities, and the extent of migration (Andorka, Cseh-Szombathy and Vavró, 1968; Farkasinszky, Ónody, Bácskai, Fodor and Szilárd, 1979; Hatvani, 1969; Moksony, 1986). Szabolcs-Szatmár County, which has undergone a strong population outflow in recent decades, was sixteenth in rank as to suicide rate (among eighteen counties) in 1950, while in 1984 it had jumped to third place.

As in most European countries, in Hungary, too, the suicide rate among the Protestant segment of the population used to be higher than among Roman Catholics. This situation changed after 1945. The suicide rate began to grow mainly in areas with predominantly Roman Catholic populations to the extent that in their suicide rate Catholics first reached then surpassed the Protestants after 1960. The contributing factors may be that a relatively larger number of Catholics live in counties with hamlets and farms where migration is particularly extensive (Böszörményi, 1977).

The suicide rate among Hungary's small Greek Catholic minority is low, which means that the Serbian and Romanian national minorities also figure low in the statistics. It may be assumed that the same applies to Hungary's Jewish population. However, the suicide rate among the ethnic Germans, the largest national minority in Hungary, is high, although no accurate statistics are available.

The breakdown according to family status follows the rates of other countries. In declining order, it is as follows: those widowed, divorced, single, and married; and the picture is the same according to age groups as well. In Hungary, too, childless couples are a higher risk group than those with children.

In terms of means employed in suicide, pills and insecticides are being increasingly used, but hanging is still very widespread. This indicates that a significant percentage of those wishing to commit suicide are of serious intent, strongly motivated and tend to be resolute. In this regard there is a difference in comparison with other countries. In Hungary, violent means of suicide are especially prevalent in the rural regions.

The statistical breakdown according to months and days of the week also shows correspondence with that of other countries. The suicide rate is higher among those with less education and among those who are in low-income categories. Many unskilled and casual labourers commit suicide. This may be related to their increased intake of alcohol. Hungary also ranks high in world statistics on alcohol consumption. The high suicide rate is also linked to the high number of alcoholics in the country. Alcoholism figures in one-third of the male suicides and is a growing factor in female suicides.

There are approximately 2–2.5 times as many men committing suicide as women in Hungary. In 1984, this figure was 2.6 yet Hungary's female population has a higher suicide rate than most other European countries. The gender bias is long standing. The discrepancy is greater in smaller communities: for example, in Budapest this index is only 1.5. In other words, compared with male suicides, female suicide in Hungary is more obviously an urban phenomenon.

Hungary's cultural heritage tends towards greater understanding and acceptance of suicide. Numerous outstanding politicians, writers, poets, and artists in Hungary have taken their own life. This has often given rise to romantic cults and legends; their example exerts an influence through history and literature classes in the schools, the message being that in certain situations suicide is an acceptable solution.

By way of example, let me mention Attila József, perhaps the greatest Hungarian poet of the twentieth century. In the last years of his life, József suffered from acute schizophrenia and in December 1937 threw himself in front of a train at Balatonszárszó. To this day, several suicides occur each year at the village station or its vicinity—this was reinforced in 1977 at the same spot by the suicide of one of Hungary's greatest actors, Zoltán Latinovits, who may be likened to the American James Dean as a cult figure.

The role of tradition is only one explanatory factor in the mystery of Hungary's high suicide rate. Another is the social anomie that set in after the Second World War, especially in the wake of the changes of 1948–9 which led to the weakening and disintegration of communities.

Preventive social mechanisms fail to operate to a sufficient degree in Hungary because social networks and support systems are underdeveloped compared with other countries. Since community support is weaker, individuals in crisis more readily fall into a presuicidal state from which relatively fewer manage escape without parasuicide and many do end their own lives.

Following the Second World War, a two-phased induced anomie came about in Hungary. The first phase was between 1948 and 1960, and the second was in the post-1960 period. This process had begun already during the War, when the attendant dislocations, refugee migrations from the battle zones and then from the Red Army, the persecution of the Jews and their mass murder, the prisoner of war camps, etc., had led to the death of many hundreds of thousands of Hungarians and contributed significantly to the disintegration of the nation's social community structure (Hankiss, 1979).

The War was followed by a period of reconstruction, and in 1948–9 came the introduction of the period called the 'building of socialism'. Upon taking power the Communist Party assumed the task of destroying the former social structure. Sociologically this meant a rapid pace of industrialisation, and Hungary soon ceased to be a predominantly agricultural country. Agricultural workers were siphoned off into the industrial sector and many became urban dwellers as a result.

The 1950s also saw the collectivisation of agriculture, which meant that millions of individually farming peasants became collective farm-workers. Migration and social mobility accelerated as hundreds of thousands changed domicile and moved vertically on the social scale. The importance of the family declined, with many of its functions supplanted by state and social institutions. Many social groups, associations, etc. were simply shut down. The political measures introduced succeeded in corroding interpersonal confidence. The spiritual and organisational role of the churches was also reduced significantly.

The accumulation of social dissatisfaction eventually led to the 1956 Revolution, following which the Communist Party had to take into account pervasive social opposition. After the initial period of organised reprisals by the new government, beginning in the 1960s a greater consumer leeway was afforded the population. The impoverished populace, deprived of all hope for political change, eagerly seized the opportunity. However, higher income was possible only at the expense of leisure time and under strong competition. This meant that what in itself was—or would have been—a positive development also exercised a negative influence on the micro-communities and covert social functions including those pertaining to mental hygiene. This was the second phase referred to above. Paradoxically, the latter proved more ruinous for the communities than the first phase, that of the overt repression of the 1950s.

What sort of communities were weakened or dissolved in post-war Hungary? The transformation from extended to nuclear families was completed, which weakened the ties of coexistence and also led to generally loosened family ties both in urban and rural parts of the country.

Workplace groups show an equivocal picture. In the case of women entering the work-force in large numbers there was increased bonding between the individual and group but at the expense of the former's relationship to family kinship relations. Residential communities experienced an unequivocal weakening of social solidarity. This was linked to urbanisation, especially since the process was so closely related to purely economic considerations. Urbanisation undermined community ties—integration in the average Hungarian town is weaker than in the villages, but the fabric has been worn thin generally.

Groups related to leisure time activities have also shown losses. With the increased opportunity for self-exploitation that began in the 1960s, people had less spare time and it must be pointed out that due to the repressive measures introduced in 1948–9, objective conditions also militated against such collectives. For example, workers choirs, which were organised by the Social Democratic Party, or the Catholic boys' and girls' were all disbanded.

Religious communities underwent a serious loss of cohesion. A twofold secularisation took place in Hungary after 1945: a spontaneous one accompanying modernisation and the one induced from above through anti-clerical campaigns. The weakening of religious or church-related communities had a significantly greater impact on the elderly, who are generally more lonely than others in any case.

Summary

In summary, it can be said that Hungary has such a high suicide rate because social integration is weaker than it should be, while anomie is strong. The leadership of the country bears a major responsibility for this because partly directly (by deliberately destroying existing communities) and partly indirectly (through consciously planned measures with negative side effects obliquely impacting on community functions) it has significantly contributed to the prevalent social anomie and high suicide rate.

Since 1968 Hungary has continued to lead the world in terms of suicide rate. In 1986, the rate was 45.3, while in second-place Denmark it was 30.3. Regarding sociological parameters, Hungary's suicides in part correspond to those of other countries (a preponderance of elderly, males, and singles; distribution according to months and days of the week), while in other respects they show divergence (higher risk among rural agricultural population; greater frequency among Catholics than Protestants; brutal means employed).

The mystery of Hungary's suicide rate is explained by two phenomena, which are complex in themselves. One is the traditional acceptance of suicide and the other is the anomie that has become pervasive in Hungarian society since 1945, the most characteristic manifestation of which is the debilitation and disintegration of communities.

References

Andorka, R. *et al.* (1986). Társadalmi beilleszkedési zavarok Magyarországon (*Social Adaptation Disorders in Hungary*), Budapest: Kossuth.

——, Cseh-Szombathy, L. and Vavró, I. (1968). 'Társadalmi elítélés alá eső magatartások előfordulásának területi különbségei' ('Regional Differences of Behaviour Types Producing Social Disapproval'), *Statisztikai Szemle*, 46, 43–54, 145–58.

Böszörményi, E. (1977). 'Az öngyilkosságok Magyarországon. Történeti és vallásszociológiai vizsgálat' ('Suicides in Hungary: An Inquiry in History and in the Sociology of Religion'), *Confessio*, 163–74.

Cseh-Szombathy, L. (1963). 'Az öngyilkosságok társadalmi jellege' ('The Social Meaning of Suicides'), *Demográfia*, 6, 186–216.

Farkasinszky, T., Ónody, S., Bácskai, M., Fodor, A. and Szilárd, J. (1979). 'Adatok az öngyilkosság-gyakoriság szociológiai okairól Csongrád megyében' ('Facts about the Sociological Causes of Suicides in the County Csongrád'), *Népegészségügy*, 60, 291–6.

Hankiss, E. (1979). 'Közösségek válsága és hiánya' ('The Crisis and Lack of Communities'), in E. Hankiss (ed.), *Társadalmi csapdák: Diagnózisok* (*Social Pitfalls: Diagnoses*), Budapest, Magvető.

Hatvani, D. (1969). 'Villámsújtottak: A Bács-Kiskún megyei öngyilkosságokról' ('People Struck by Lightening: About the Suicides in Bács-Kiskún County'), *Forrás*, 5–6, 51–63.

Jobb, S. (1973). 'Az öngyilkosság területi jellemzői Magyarországon' ('About the Regional Characteristics of Suicides in Hungary'), *Területi Statisztika*, 23, 39–53.

Moksony, F. (1986). 'Települési tényezők és öngyilkosság' ('Settlement Factors and Suicides'), in B. Buda and J. Füredi (eds.), *Az öngyilkosság a szociálpszichiátria szempontjából* (*The Suicide from the Point of View of Social Psychiatry*), Budapest: Magyar Pszichiátriai Társaság.

Szigeti, P. (1986). 'Az öngyilkosságok alakulása Magyarországon a hatvanas évek elejétől napjainkig a főbb demográfiai szempontok szerint' ('Suicides in Hungary from the Beginnings of the 1960s to our Days from the Point of View of the Chief Demographic Characteristics'), in B. Buda and J. Füredi (eds.), *Az öngyilkosság a szociálpszichiátria szempontjából* (*The Suicide from the Point of View of Society Psychiatry*), Budapest: Magyar Pszichiátriai Társaság.

Changes in the Irish suicide rate

M.J. KELLEHER and M. DALY

The Irish suicide rates have always been an enigma and of great epidemiological interest. Here was an island population of similar language and cultural history situated close to Britain but publicly recording a suicide rate which, in 1960, was only one-quarter of that recorded in England and Wales. This low Irish suicide rate provoked disbelief. Two studies, one carried out in the 1960s (McCarthy and Walsh, 1975) and one in early 1980s (Clarke Finnegan and Fahy, 1983) indicated that Irish coroners were under-recording suicide verdicts when individual cases were reassessed by the investigating authors.

The question not investigated, however, in this regard was whether Irish coroners, as a group, were more likely to under-record suicide verdicts than coroners from Britain. Two British studies strongly suggested that unreliability between coroners was not likely to be the main explanation why national figures differed. The first of these studies was by Barraclough (1970), who found that there were no significant differences between two sets of coroners' districts in the rate in which suicide was recorded when, in one set, the coroner had remained the same in the two periods of study, while in the other set, the coroners had changed. The second study was by Ross and Kreitman (1975), who found that when the typescript of evidence in cases of possible suicide was exchanged between coroners in England and Wales on the one hand with similar officials in Scotland on the other, whereas there might be disagreement in individual cases, the overall trend remained the same. This strongly implied that the official statistics, in spite of their many shortcomings, are valid for cross-national comparison.

The strongest evidence in favour of a low Irish suicide rate

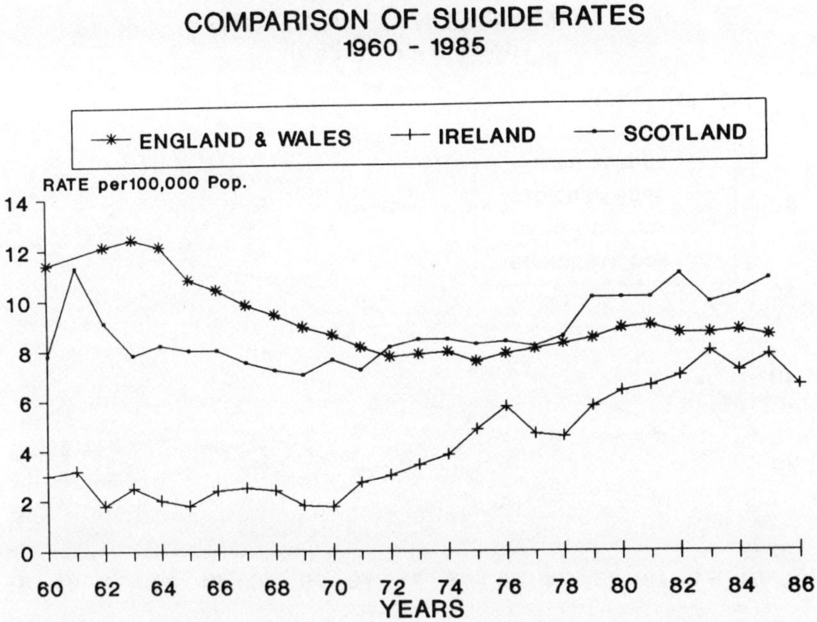

Figure 1: Comparison of suicide rates for Ireland, Scotland, England and Wales 1960–85) taken from WHO Yearbooks)

throughout the 1960s (Figure 1) is provided by Sainsbury (1973). He showed that when the Irish statistics on suicide are compared with those from eleven other countries, the Irish rate is the second lowest, lying tenth in rank order. When the suicide statistics for the United States of America are examined by immigrant groups, the Irish rate, although higher than those at home, still retains the same rank order, remaining second lowest in the tenth position. It must be concluded that the Irish suicide rate was genuinely very low.

The second reason why the suicide rate in Ireland is of great epidemiological interest is that over the past fourteen years there has been a very marked increase in suicide (Figure 1), which demands a definitive explanation. The present work is an attempt to clarify this problem.

Between 1970 and 1985, there has been approximately a sixfold increase in the annual numbers of individual cases of suicide recorded in the Republic of Ireland. It is a matter of the first importance to determine whether this increase is genuine or whether it is simply a change in recording practice. If it were simply a change in recording practice, then, as the official

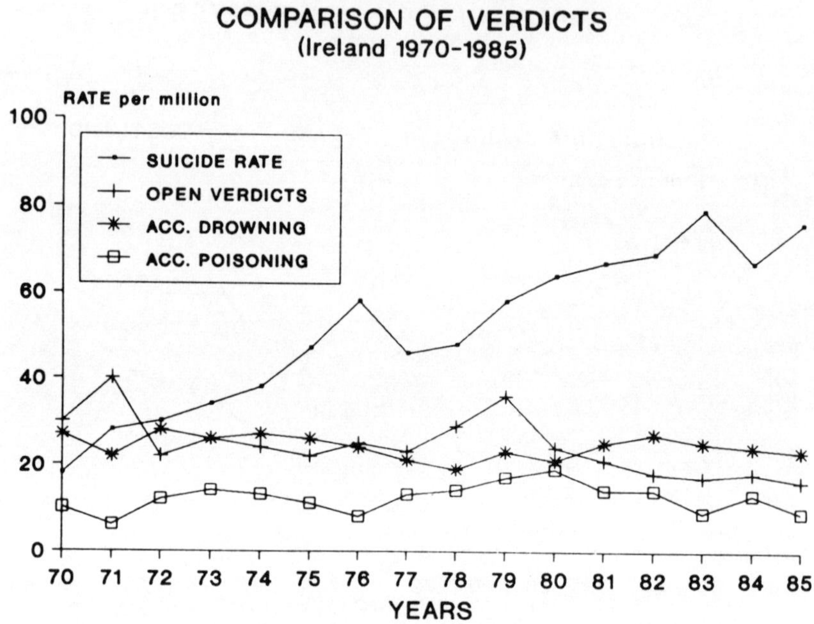

Figure 2: Comparison of verdicts (Ireland 1970–85)

numbers of suicides increase there would be a concomitant fall in the numbers of accidental drowning, accidental poisoning, and cases where an open verdict was recorded. As Figure 2 shows, this is clearly not the case. In other words the increase is genuine.

Age has a big influence on rates of suicide. The usual pattern is for the suicide rate to increase in each decade from the second decade onwards up to the seventh decade when there is a rapid fall off. The Irish rates, particularly amongst men (Figure 3) do not follow this pattern, in contrast to England and Wales.

The major increase in suicide rates has been in the early and middle-years with a sharp fall off in the fifth decade. The explanation for this demands further investigation. One possibility is that the Irish elderly and late middle-aged are set in their ways and secure in their value systems which protects them emotionally from the rapid secular changes in Irish society. Another possibility, discussed later, is that the young and middle-aged are most vulnerable to the consequences of sudden and unexpected unemployment.

It is a perennial question as to whether those who take their lives by suicide are mentally ill in the weeks before death. It is not

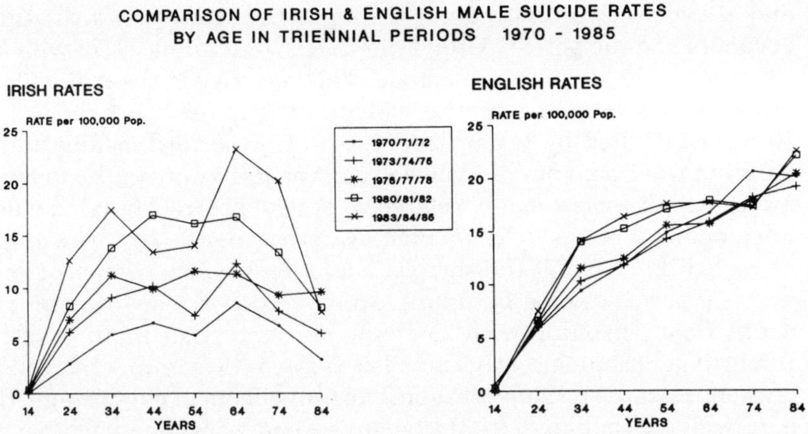

Figure 3: Comparison of Irish and English male suicide rates, by age in triennial periods (1979–85)

necessary that they should be so, particularly in those cultures which counsel or encourage suicide under particular circumstances. In Western, and in societies of Christian origin in particular, suicide has been regarded as a taboo act which attracts social and moral prohibition involving dire consequences for the good name of the individual and the well-being of his family. Under these circumstances it is hardly surprising that those who take their lives by suicide have come to be regarded as being mentally ill at the time of death. One study of a hundred cases of suicide (Barraclough *et al.* 1974) found that approximately 90 per cent suffered from either depression or alcoholism prior to death. It does not necessarily follow from this, however, that at times of rapid social change, when there is a great increase in the suicide rate, that all those who take their lives are mentally ill in the ordinary clinical meaning of the term.

There is no evidence from official Irish hospital statistics to indicate a change in frequency of mental illness which would explain the increase in suicide rate. The most likely interpretation is that a depressed Irish man or woman of today is much more likely to consider suicide as a way out of difficult circumstances than their counterparts of, say, twenty years ago. But why is there this marked change in attitude?

Before endeavouring to answer this question, reference must be made to the methods used to terminate life. They are characterised, particularly amongst men, by being both punitive and unpleasant. Each case of suicide occurring in Cork between 1980 and 1985, was investigated through consultation with the coroners and the police. Altogether there were 207 cases, of which 149 were male and 58 were female. The majority of the men (103) either drowned or hanged themselves, only 15 (or approximately 10 per cent) died by taking overdoses of prescribed medication; hanging was commoner in rural areas and drowning in the urban areas, which was probably related to ease of access. Hanging was uncommon amongst the women, whereas death by drowning occurred in over half the sample. Eighteen women, or approximately 30 per cent, died by taking drug overdoses. The low rate of death from poisoning with medicine merits further inquiry, particularly as so much costly emphasis is given to avoiding tricyclic anti-depressants because of their harmful effects in overdosage. It may well be that lives could be saved had tricyclic drugs been given more frequently in adequate dosages in appropriate cases.

If it is accepted that the Irish suicide rate was previously low and is now genuinely much higher comparable to other European countries, and that there has been no concomitant dramatic change in illness patterns, then clearly the increased suicide rate must be sought in the social and psychological sphere. It is an unclear and speculative area where fortunately one can benefit from the work done by others.

Durkheim's work (1897) implies that society determines its own rate of suicide. Among the factors which in other countries have been found to correlate highly with the suicide rate have been the crime rate, the level of alcoholism, the illegitimacy rate, and the divorce rate. Taken together these disparate rates may be seen as representing the level of integration or cohesion within society, as the work of Sainsbury *et al.* (1980) outlines.

The Irish illegitimacy rates which were taken from the *Report on Vital Statistics* (Central Statistics Office Dublin, 1970–83) show that there was an increase in illegitimacy in each succeeding year beginning in 1970 with a rate of 5.7 per 1000 unmarried females aged 15–49 and ending in 1983 at 12.7 per 1000 unmarried females (Figure 4). The numbers of indictable crimes were taken from the *Report on Crime* published by the Irish Police (Garda Siochana, 1985) and show that between 1975 and 1985 the numbers of indictable offences doubled, rising from 48 387 to 91 285. Two measures of alcoholism were used. The consumption of alcohol per head was taken from the *Report Produktschap Voor Gedistilleerde Drauken Schiedam Netherlands* reproduced by the Health Education Bureau Dublin (1985). The second measure of alcoholism used was

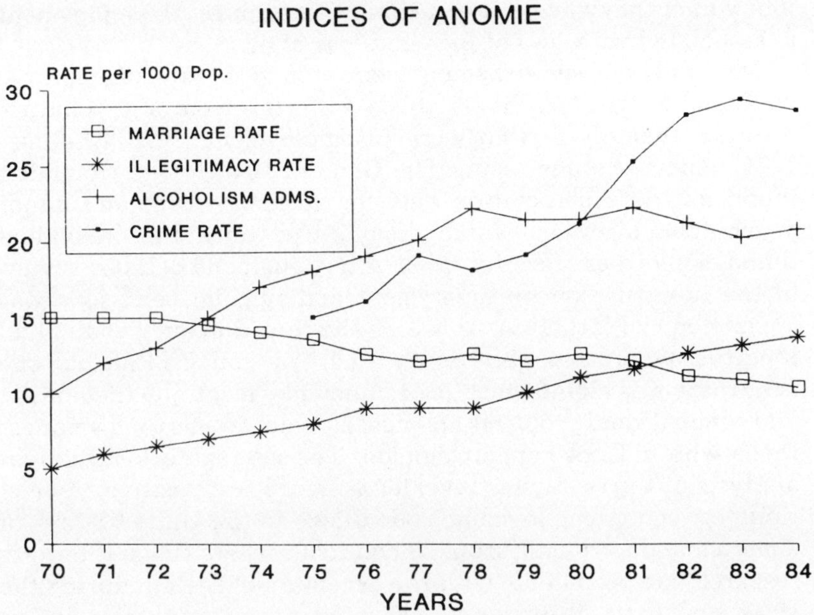

Figure 4: Indices of anomie

the number of admissions to hospital for alcoholism taken from the reports of the Medico Social Research Board (1971–83). Both these measures of possible alcoholism in Irish society showed an increase in tandem with the increase in the suicide rate. The marriage rates for different years were taken from the *Report on Vital Statistics* (Central Statistics Office, Dublin, 1971–83). Between 1971 and 1984, the Irish marriage rate fell in a step-wise fashion from 7.4 per 1000 population in 1971 to 5.8 in 1982.

Thus, these four measures—namely the illegitimacy rate, the crime rate, the alcoholism rate, and the fall in the marriage rate—confirm Sainsbury's findings in an Irish context. It does not offer a proximate causative explanation, however. At most, it suggests that the same forces which determine these changes in measures of integration and disintegration also influence the rise in suicide.

Unemployment touches the individual personally and more immediately. For well over a century, Western society has used compulsory education not only as a method of imparting literary and practical skills but also as a means to inculcate in the individual the spirit of the work ethic. Good men are men with good jobs which they have a responsibility to acquire. Unemployment is associated with loss of face and loss of prestige.

One study of some 400 young people found that the unemployed were six times more likely to be suffering from a psychiatric disorder than those who were in employment (Findlay Jones, 1984). Another study, using The General Health Questionnaire, found a strong association between unemployment and minor psychiatric disorder, which disappeared once the individual found employment (Banks, 1982). A thorough and detailed review of the literature on unemployment and suicidal behaviour was completed by Platt (1984), in which the results of eight individual longitudinal studies were reviewed. It was found in all but one that there was significantly more unemployment, job instability, and occupational problems amongst suicide victims than amongst those who did not commit suicide. The aggregate longitudinal analysis of thirty studies revealed a significant positive association between unemployment and suicide in the United States of America and various European countries where the appropriate research had been done, with the exception of Britain during the 1960s and early 1970s where there was a negative correlation which was thought to be due to the decreasing toxicity of domestic gas.

It is well known that Irish unemployment rates are very high. Of the men who took their lives in Cork, some two-thirds were out of work at the time of their death. Financial poverty per se is not related to suicide rate (Sainsbury, 1955), rather it is poverty of relationships and loss or absence of social opportunities. For many, particularly men, employment supplies a ready-made set of relationships, offering the individual a sense of purpose, obligation, and reciprocal support outside the domestic unit. Loss of this sense of belonging possibly disposes towards suicide.

Roman Catholicism is the stated religion of more than 95 per cent of the population of the Republic of Ireland. Unlike the Protestant religions with their doctrine of the elect, Catholics traditionally remain loyal to the medieval doctrine of the four last things—namely Death, Judgement, Heaven, and Hell—or, in other words, the manner of one's death determined one's disposition in the next life. In recent years, the sway of traditional Catholic values has waned, particularly amongst the young as is reflected in falling church attendance and attendance at the sacraments. Death by suicide is no longer so great a taboo. The notoriety given to the suicides of well-known personages has added to this change in attitude. Contagion of behaviour is a factor; within Cork a particular bridge over the River Lee became the site of a series of suicides among young men all known personally to each other. Perhaps secular materialism per se is less adequate than traditional cultural values in providing the distressed with reasons for living.

In conclusion, earlier Irish suicide rates were probably genuinely low, but there has been a marked increase over the past fifteen years so that the true Irish suicide rates are now comparable with other Western European countries. This increase in the suicide rate is not due to changes in the frequency of psychiatric illnesses. Three sets of social and psychological changes may have contributed to this increase. These changes include measures of a loss of social integration; increasing unemployment; and loss of traditional spiritual values with the increasing secularisation of Irish society.

References

Banks, M.H. and Jackson, P.R. (1982). 'Unemployment and Risk of Minor Psychiatric Disorder in Young People—Cross Sectional and Longitudinal Evidence', *Psychological Medicine*, 12, 789–98.

Barraclough, B. (1970). The effect that coroners have on the suicide rate and the open verdict rate. In: *Psychiatric Epidemiology*. Eds. E.A. Hare and J.K. Wing.

Barraclough, B.M., Bunch, J., Nelson, B. and Sainsbury, P. (1974). A Hundred Cases of Suicide—Clinical Aspects', *British Journal of Psychiatry*, 125, 355–73.

Clarke, F.M. and Fahy, T.J. (1983). 'Suicide Rates in Ireland', *Psychological Medicine*, 13, 385–91.

Durkheim, E. (1897). *Le Suicide*, translated (1952) as *Suicide: A Study Sociology* by J.A. Spaulding and C. Simpson, London: Routledge & Kegan Paul.

Findlay Jones, R. and Eckhardt, (1984). Survey of Unemployment Among Young People', *Australian & New Zealand Journal of Psychiatry*, 18, 135–43.

Medico Social Research Board, *Activities of Irish Psychiatric Hospitals 1971–1983.*

McCarthy, D. and Walsh, D. (1975). 'The Under-Reporting of Suicide and the Consequences for National Statistics', *British Journal of Psychiatry*, 126, 301–8.

Platt, S. (1984). 'Unemployment and Suicidal Behaviour—A Review of Literature, *Social Science and Medicine*, 19 (2), 93–115.

Produktschap Voor Gedistilleerde Drauken Schiedam Netherlands (1985), reproduced by Health Education Bureau, Dublin.

Report on Crime 1983, 1984, 1985, the Garda Siochana, 3.

Report on Vital Statistics CSO 1970–1985, Table XIV: Births per 1000 Women in Each Age Group, Ireland and England & Wales.

Report on Vital Statistics 1971–1985, Table 1: 'Number of Marriages per 1000 Population in Ireland and Neighbouring Countries'.

Ross, O. and Kreitman, N. (1975). 'A Further Investigation of Differences in the Suicide Rate of England & Wales and of Scotland', *British Journal of Psychiatry*, 127, 575–82.

Sainsbury, P. (1955). *Suicide in London*, Maudsley Monograph No. 1, London: Chapman & Hall.

——(1973). 'Suicide: Opinions and Facts', *Proc. Roy. Soc. Med.*, 66, 579–87.

——, Jenkins, J. and Levey, A. (1980). 'The Social Correlates of Suicide in Europe', in R.D.T. Farmer and S.R. Hirsch (eds.), *The Suicide Syndrome*, London: Croom Helm.

2

SOCIAL FACTORS AND SUICIDE

Unemployment and mortality in Italy: the Turin longitudinal study

G. COSTA, P. CREPET and F. FLORENZANO

Unemployment and suicide in Italy

Various researchers have examined the links between unemployment and suicide, and the subject has received particular attention as a result of a labour market crisis which has made jobs increasingly difficult to find in all industrialised countries (Barraclough *et al.* 1974; Platt, 1984; Pritchard, 1988). However, few studies have been able to examine the unemployment–suicide link at the individual level (Humphrey, 1977; Shepherd and Barraclough, 1980; Hagnell and Rorsman, 1980).

Unemployment levels in Italy show no signs of abating (the official figure rose to 13 per cent of the total population in 1987) and are now among the highest in Europe. As Table 1 shows,

TABLE 1: Unemployment and suicides: specific rates of unemployment and suicides by sex, Italy, Trend 1978–87

	Unemployment rate/100			*Suicide rate/100 000*		
Year	*M*	*F*	*MF*	*M*	*F*	*MF*
1978	4.7	12.6	7.2	6.8	2.5	4.7
1979	4.9	13.3	7.7	6.7	2.6	4.7
1980	4.8	13.1	7.6	6.6	2.7	4.7
1981	5.4	14.4	8.4	7.2	2.6	4.9
1982	6.1	14.9	9.1	7.5	2.9	5.2
1983	6.6	16.2	9.9	7.2	2.9	5.0
1984	6.8	17.1	10.0	8.2	3.1	5.6
1985	7.0	17.3	10.3	9.5	3.5	6.4
1986	7.4	17.8	11.1	9.5	3.7	6.6
1987	8.1	18.7	12.0	10.6	4.1	7.3

Source: ISTAT

TABLE 2: Suicide rate (per 100 000) among employed and unemployed (in search of the 1st and of a new employment), 1978–87

	A			*B*			*C*			*B + C*		
	Employed			*In search of 1st employment*			*In search of new employment*			*Unemployed*		
Year	*M*	*F*	*MF*	*M*	*F*	*MF*	*M*	*F*	*MF*	*M*	*F*	*MF*
1978	6.0	2.5	4.9	9.6	1.2	5.3	8.8	0.6	3.8	9.3	0.9	4.6
1979	6.4	2.2	5.1	5.8	1.5	3.6	13.9	1.0	5.9	9.3	1.2	4.7
1980	6.1	1.7	5.0	9.7	0.8	5.1	25.8	2.5	11.0	16.4	1.7	7.8
1981	6.5	1.7	5.0	8.5	1.5	4.8	20.5	1.2	8.4	13.6	1.4	6.5
1982	6.7	1.9	5.2	6.3	1.0	3.5	26.1	2.0	11.6	13.6	1.4	6.5
1983	5.6	1.6	4.3	4.7	0.6	2.6	25.7	3.5	12.3	12.9	2.0	6.8
1984	6.5	1.8	5.0	6.9	1.9	4.3	25.7	2.0	11.0	15.6	2.0	7.7
1985	7.2	1.9	5.5	7.9	1.4	4.5	34.0	1.8	14.2	21.5	1.4	10.0
1986	7.2	2.1	5.5	11.5	1.2	6.1	32.3	2.6	13.8	20.8	1.9	10.0
1987	7.2	1.8	5.4	13.8	7.8	10.8	33.2	2.9	14.5	22.7	5.1	12.7

Source: ISTAT

increasing unemployment parallels the greater risk of death by suicide for both sexes in the population as a whole.

Legal statistics are themselves a possible source for analysis of the risk of death by suicide according to occupational status (Table 2). In the case of the unemployed the raw mortality rates for suicide consistently stand at around double the value for the unemployed in search of new jobs. Among women suicide-related mortality rates do not vary appreciably with variations in occupational status (Crepet and Florenzano, 1988).

However, the Italian legal sources for statistics on suicide (ISTAT) are incomplete, since not all suicides are reported and there is no way of assessing the reliability of the coverage. Furthermore, the data issued by this source cannot be standardised according to age.

The only alternative open to us would be to use the ISTAT *mortality* statistics, since they cover all cases and the data published are broken down according to age groups. Unfortunately, however, these statistics are not presented in terms of occupational status and, therefore, cannot be drawn on for a nationwide analysis of mortality rate relating to suicide among the unemployed.

Mortality among the unemployed: the Turin Longitudinal Study

In Turin, a city in the north-east region of Italy with a population of over 2 million inhabitants, a survey system has been introduced which offers data on the suicide risk according to occupational status, and we shall, therefore, refer to this context in our attempt to verify at the individual level the hypothesis of an increased mortality risk for violent causes and accidents (mostly suicides) among the unemployed seeking new jobs.

The Turin Longitudinal Study was achieved by matching registry office records with census records (1981 ISTAT population census) on an individual basis. Thus, a number of significant demographic elements (death, marriage, birth of a child) subsequent to the census are added to the personal census records of individuals still resident in the city. If subjects emigrate, their continued survival is periodically verified. This contribution applies to mortality due to violent causes and accidents for resident subjects of working age (men 15–59; women 15–54) according to the occupational status declared in the census.

The mortality ratio standardised according to age (SMR) was used as a convenient index of mortality: it yields the ratio between the number of deaths observed and the number expected (× 100) in the study group. Mortality expectations were obtained by applying the specific mortality rates for age (five-year groups) relating to a standard reference population (in this case the population selected) to the number of person-years at risk in the study group (e.g. the unemployed). The 95 per cent two-tailed confidence limits for the SMR were calculated using Poisson's distribution for observed deaths.

Results and discussion

The study included 13 462 males aged 15–59 who were unemployed and, according to their census statements, in search of a new job. During the period 1981–85 this group showed general mortality levels twice as high as the expected levels (SMR = 202, CL 95 per cent 179–227, 284 observed deaths). This excess risk applied to practically all the major categories of causes of death, showing peaks for accidental or violent causes (SMR = 244, CL 95 per cent 187–313, 61 observed deaths).

Table 3 shows specific mortality due to the main types of accidental and violent causes. Representation of all the categories of external causes of death is significantly above expectation levels, with the exception of accidents involving means of transport.

TABLE 3: Mortality among the unemployed seeking new jobs according to type of external cause, Turin, 1981–5

Type of Cause (ICD E)	*SMR*	*Observed deaths*	*CL 95%*
Accidents involving means of transport (800–848)	145	13	77–250
Accidental poisoning (850–869)	318	5	103–742
Suicide (950–959)	285	15	159–470
Murder (960–979)	682	9	311–1294
Other types	241	19	145–376

Accidental poisoning (five deaths) is entirely represented by cases of heroin overdose.

It has been objected that the unemployed lose their jobs (thus undergoing selection) because they are less healthy or more prone to conditions entailing a greater death risk. If this were indeed the case, then the risk should reach a peak around the time of selection (near to the census point); with the passing of time and the death of more susceptible people the risk level should drop towards expectation levels. However, Table 4 shows that the true trend in accidental and violent deaths is exactly the opposite, and this would seem partly to rule out the selection effect. This also applies to suicides.

The only category of accidental causes to show a striking peak at the beginning of the follow-up is the category 'other types', including a number of deaths due to falls in the home in the case of alcoholics, for example. This is a reasonable sign of a residual selection of prone subjects among the unemployed.

Analysis of mortality according to the combinations of occupa-

TABLE 4: Mortality due to accidental or violent causes among the unemployed seeking new jobs, according to calendar year

Calender year	*SMR*	*Observed deaths*	*CL 95%*
1981–2	91	6	33–198
1983	220	13	117–376
1984	288	18	171–455
1985	388	24	249–577

TABLE 5: Mortality due to accidental or violent causes or suicide according to occupational status held in 1976 and 1981

Occupational status *1976*	*1981*	*Accidental and violent causes SMR (obs)*	*Suicides SMR (obs)*
empl.	empl.	83 (301)*	82 (81)*
unempl.	empl.	91 (9)	129 (3)
empl.	unempl.	210 (21)*	318 (8)*
unempl.	unempl.	451 (27)*	363 (5)*

(*) p < = 0.05.

tional status experienced in 1976 and 1981, as referred to 1981 census (Table 5) demonstrates that the risk of violent or accidental death or suicide is significantly higher in the case of subjects who lost their jobs between 1976 and 1981, and rises even higher for the long-term unemployed. Therefore, the risk appears to increase when unemployment persists.

An alternative explanation might be that the social class distribution of the unemployed differs from that of the population as a whole. The lower social classes are, in fact, marked by a higher mortality risk, and it is precisely these classes that are represented among the unemployed.

In Table 6 mortality resulting from accidental and violent causes is analysed specifically according to status as home occupier and level of education taken as indicators of social class. The risk remains appreciably high in each of the groups concerned; and the SMR standardised according to home occupier status stand at 237 for accidental and violent deaths and 278 for suicides.

One further point worth noting is that among women of

TABLE 6: Mortality due to accidental and violent causes and suicide among the unemployed according to type of home occupancy and level of education

Variable	*Accidental or violent causes SMR (obs)*	*Suicides SMR (obs.)*
Own house	334 (17)*	448 (5)*
Rented house	223 (40)*	248 (9)*
Education: degree/ advanced level	311 (9)*	
ordinary/ lower level	181 (19)	
elementary or otherwise	261 (33)*	

(*) < = 0.05.

working age the SMR for subjects seeking employment (first and new, about 25 049 subjects) stands at 125, based on 83 observed deaths (CL 95 per cent 100–56). Despite the scantiness of these findings, this slight excess in mortality can, in part, be accounted for by an appreciable suicide risk (9 observed against an expectation of 3.16, SMR = 284, CL 95 per cent 130–541), comparable to the risk level ascertained among males.

Furthermore, it is found among young people who have never had a job and who were looking for work at the last census (9946 boys and 13 879 girls) that there is a significant excess death rate due to accidental and violent causes (male SMR = 145, 32 observed deaths, CL 95 per cent 99–205; female SMR = 176, 18 observed deaths, CL 95 per cent = 104–277). These excesses can be partly explained by eleven deaths due to drug overdose (six males, five females), compared with three expected cases of accidental poisoning.

In conclusion, the Turin Longitudinal Study reveals that the risk of death due to accidental or violent causes among males (including suicide and comparable accidental death, e.g. drug overdose) who have lost their jobs and are seeking new ones is double the risk for the rest of the Turin population of the same age. This finding is confirmed by results regarding unemployed women.

The increased risk does not appear to be an effect of the selection of the subjects prone to accidental or violent death among the unemployed. Moreover, the risk increases as unemployment is protracted, and this cannot be attributed to the different age and social class distribution that distinguish the unemployed from the rest of population.

Finally, this risk pattern tallies in structure and degree with a similar pattern emerging from initial analyses of mortality among the English unemployed between 1981 and 1983 (Moser *et al.* 1987). We may, therefore, reasonably suppose that unemployment plays a role, albeit a possibly indirect one, in the formation of the risk pattern.

References

Barraclough, B., Bunch, J., Nelson, B. and Sainsbury, P. (1974). 'A Hundred Cases of Suicide: Clinical Aspects', *British J. Psychiatry*, 125, 355–73.

Crepet, P. and Florenzano, F. (1988). 'Suicide and Unemployment in Italy', in H.J. Moller, A. Schmidtke and R. Welz (eds.), *Current Issues of Suicidology*, Berlin: Springer-Verlag.

Hagnell, O. and Rorsman, B. (1980). 'Suicide in the Lundby Study: A Controlled Prospective Investigation of Stressful Life Events', *Neuropsychobiology*, 6, 319–32.

Humphrey, J. (1977). 'Social Loss: A Comparison of Suicide Victims, Homicide Offenders and Non-Violent Individuals', *Dis. Nerv. Syst.*, 38, 157–60.

Moser, K.A., Goldblatt, P.O., Fox, A.J. and Jones, D.R. (1987). 'Unemployment and Mortality: Comparison of the 1971 and 1981 Longitudinal Study Census Samples', *British Medical J.*, 294, 86–90.

Platt, S. (1984) 'Unemployment and Suicidal Behaviour: A Review of the Literature', *Soc. Sci. Med.*, 2, 93–115.

Pritchard, C. (1988). 'Suicide, Unemployment and Gender in the British Isles and European Community (1974–1985)', *Social Psychiatry*, 23, 85–9.

Shepard, D.M. and Barraclough, B.M. 1980). 'Work and Suicide: An Empirical Investigation', *British J. Psychiatry*, 136, 469–78.

Suicidal drive in urban and rural communities of North Italy: a comparison

D. DE LEO, D. BANON, F. SCHIFANO, M. VASCON and L. PAVAN

Introduction

In recent years the incidence of suicide, and especially of attempted suicide, has increased notably in many European countries (WHO, 1982, Diekstra, 1985). In Italy, according to official statistics, the incidence of suicide is low and that of attempted suicide very low (ISTAT, 1980–5). However, even in Italy there has been an appreciable increase in suicide mortality since 1975 (from 5.6 per 100 000 inhabitants in 1975 to 6.8 in 1980), while officials statistics show a reduction in attempted suicides. Our institute has implemented an epidemiological study to evaluate the real incidence of suicidal behaviour in the city of Padua. This study has revealed that the frequency of suicide is probably 100 per cent higher than reported in the national statistics, while that of attempted suicide is 10–15 times higher (De Leo *et al.* 1987, 1988).

As part of a research programme on the real incidence of suicidal behaviour in the Veneto region (in which our city is located), we set up a series of studies in rural areas around Padua in order to build a 'map' of suicidal behaviour in the region. Interest in this type of survey in Italy in general derives from the need for more reliable data than those provided by the National Institute of Statistics (ISTAT) which, for 1985, for example, reported 1 826 cases of attempted suicide for the whole country as against 3 706 suicides (ISTAT, 1980–5). Figures of this sort require no further comment; it is reasonable to presume that the real figures for attempted suicide may be at least 15–20 times higher (De Leo *et al.* 1988). Obviously, the problem of underestimation of suicidal behaviour is not confined to Italy but is a tendency in every country, as noted by the WHO (1982). It goes without saying that the characteristics and magnitude of the underestimation will vary from country to country.

In the study presented here we felt that it would be useful to compare suicidal patterns in rural and urban areas. Such a comparison may also help to reveal the existence of specific risk factors for a particular area, the identification of which may provide the basis for preventive action in relation to suicidal behaviour (Jacobson and Reuberg, 1985).

A further aim of this study is to compare data on the incidence of suicide and attempted suicide in Padua with data relating to the Veneto health catchment area (ULSS) No. 18, which includes nine local authority areas between Padua and Venice.

Materials and methods

The 1981 census gave the population of the city of Padua as 234 674. The ULSS No. 18 catchment area includes nine local authorities with a total population on 31 December 1983 of 99 533. The socio-economic structure of this area is basically agricultural, but there are also numerous and predominantly family-run small and medium business concerns.

Suicides

In Italy there are two sources of information on suicides. One is the data collected by the civil and military law enforcement agencies (police and *carabinierei*) in the case of all deaths not due to natural causes. These data are collated by the government statistics office (ISTAT) and published in the *Italian Statistical Yearbook.* The other source is given by medical death statistics, collected by the registrar's office of each local authority and periodically sent to ISTAT, which publishes them in the *Yearbook of Health Statistics.* Cecere and Florenzano (1984) compared the two publications, finding that the *Italian Statistical Yearbook* reported a number of cases averaging 10–15 per cent lower than that given by the *Yearbook of Health Statistics.* However, we gathered our data on suicides in the study area from the registers held at the *carabinieri* stations, as the death certificate data collated by the various local authorities proved unreliable. (According to this source a mere seven suicides occurred during the period under consideration. This was why, as we shall see later, we were obliged to use two different methods of data collection for the two samples.) We considered suicides registered between 1

May 1982 and 1 May 1986 in the seven *carabinieri* stations serving the nine local authority areas. Thirty-three subjects (twenty-eight males and five females) were identified. Socio-demographic data and modality of suicide were considered for each subject. Other data were not available.

In Padua, we considered all suicides committed by city residents over the same period and registered at the city registrar's office. One hundred and seven subjects (sixty-two males and forty-five females) were identified. Socio-demographic characteristics and suicidal method were compared with the data for suicides among the residents of ULSS No. 18.

Attempted suicides

Due to the unreliability of official statistics on attempted suicides, we collected the data ourselves. We identified 235 consecutive subjects presenting at the casualty unit of the only hospital in ULSS catchment area No. 18 as a consequence of attempted suicide over the period 1 May 1982 to 1 May 1986. The examination was carried out retrospectively, based on the available records (clinical record cards for those admitted to hospital and psychiatric consultation reports for those treated only in the casualty unit of Dolo [Venice] General Hospital).

These data were compared with information relating to the 223 attempted suicides observed during 1986 among residents of the city of Padua. From a methodological point of view, we should point out that the data from the two sources were collected by different medical staffs, giving rise to the possibility of unreliable diagnoses and a variable level of accuracy in the drafting of verbal reports.

Results

Suicides

Table 1 shows the data concerning the characteristics of suicides in the two areas considered.

The mean annual incidence of suicide was 8.29 cases per 100 000 population in the local authorities served by ULSS No. 18, and 11.4 cases per 100 000 in Padua. The male–female ratio of successful suicides in the two areas were very different: 5.6 to 1 in ULSS No. 18; and 1.37 to 1 in Padua. Mean age in the two samples was, respectively, 60.2 (s.d. 19.3) and 54.8 (s.d. 16.1); 38.3 per cent of suicides in ULSS No. 18 were committed by married people, 33.4

TABLE 1: Characteristics of completed suicides (1st May 1982–1st May 1986)

	Padua	*ULSS 18*	
n	107	33	
m/f	62/45	28/5	$p < 0.01$
incidence	11.4/100.000	8.3/100.000	
mean age	54.8 (s.d. 16.1)	60.2 (s.d. 19.3	
Marital status:			
married	55.1%	38.3%	
unmarried	28.0%	28.3%	
widows/ers	14.1%	33.4%	
separated	2.8%	—	
Job occupation:			
pensioner	38.3%	54.3%	
employed	36.5%	33.5%	
unemployed	1.9%	9.2%	
housewife	18.7%	3.0%	
student	3.7%	—	
Suicidal method:			
hanging	28.9%	51.5%	
drowning	14.9%	18.2%	
defenestration	20.6%	12.1%	
firearms	9.3%	9.0%	
drug overdose	7.5%	6.1%	
moving vehicles	4.7%	3.1%	
other methods	14.5%	—	

X^2 (Yates' correction).

per cent by widows/ers, and 28.3 per cent by unmarried persons. Married people accounted for a higher percentage in Padua (55.1 per cent), and were followed by unmarried people (28 per cent), widows/ers (14.1 per cent) and separated people (2.8 per cent).

The most frequent employment status in the two populations was retired (54 per cent) in ULSS No. 18, 38.3 per cent in Padua); 36.4 per cent of the Paduan cases had regular employment as against 33 per cent in ULSS No. 18; 9.2 per cent of the ULSS No. 18 population were unemployed compared with 1.9 per cent in Padua; and 3 per cent of the ULSS No. 18 cases as against 18.7 per cent of the Paduan cases were housewives; 3.7 per cent of the Paduan population were students.

Data on schooling levels is unfortunately not comparable as this was not recorded in 66.6 per cent of the ULSS No. 18 cases.

Hanging was the most common method of suicide, especially in the ULSS No. 18 population (51.5 per cent of cases compared with 28.9 per cent in Padua). This method was followed in the ULSS No. 18 population by drowning (18.2 per cent as against 14.9 per cent in Padua). The second most frequent method in Padua was defenestration (20.6 per cent), which was the third method in order of frequency in the ULSS No. 18 population (12.1 per cent). This was followed by firearms (9 per cent in ULSS No. 18 compared with 9.3 per cent in Padua), and drug overdose (respectively, 6.1 per cent and 7.5 per cent; 3 per cent of the ULSS No. 18 and 4.7 per cent of the Paduan cases threw themselves under moving vehicles. In Padua, a further 14.5 per cent of subjects committed suicide by other methods.

Statistical analysis (chi-squared) of the data for the two populations revealed significant differences for sex distribution and marginally for marital status, widows/ers in particular being more frequent among suicides in the ULSS No. 18 population. No other statistically significant differences emerged.

Attempted suicides

Table 2 shows the characteristics of attempted suicides in the two areas considered. The mean annual incidence of attempted suicide was 59.0 per 100 000 inhabitants in the ULSS No. 18 catchment area and 92.9 in Padua. Females were more frequent in both populations: 162 subjects (64.94 per cent) in ULSS No. 18 and 133 (59.7 per cent) in Padua.

The male to female ratio was 0.45 to 1 in ULSS No. 18 and 0.67 to 1 in Padua. The mean age was 39.3 (s.d. 18.2) in ULSS No. 18 and 33.5 (s.d. 17.3) in Padua.

In ULSS No. 18 48.5 per cent of suicide attempters were married, compared with 22.5 per cent in Padua. Unmarried persons made up 47.5 per cent of the Paduan population and 39.6 per cent of the ULSS No. 18 population; 5.5 per cent of the ULSS and 6.8 per cent of the Paduan subjects were separated or divorced.

The most common employment status among the ULSS No. 18 population was 'housewife' (40.4 per cent), while this group represented only 14.8 per cent of the Paduan cases; 26.9 per cent of the Paduan subjects and 21.3 per cent of ULSS No. 18 subjects had regular employment, while the unemployed accounted for 13.5 per cent of the Paduan and 18.7 per cent of the ULSS No. 18 subjects; 12.8 per cent of ULSS No. 18 and 13.5 per cent of Paduan subjects were retired; 8.9 per cent of the Paduan group were students as against 6.82 per cent of the ULSS No. 18 group. The subject's occupation was unknown in 16.6 per cent of the Paduan subjects.

The prevalent suicidal method in both populations was drug

TABLE 2: Characteristics of attempted suicides

	Padua (1986)	*ULSS 18 (1st May 82–1st May 86)*	
N	223	235	
m/f	90/133	73/162	$p < 0.05$
incidence	92.9/100.000	59.0/100.000	$p < 0.01$
mean age	33.5 (s.d. 17.3)	39.3 (s.d. 18.2)	
Marital status:			
married	22.5%	48.5%	$p < 0.001$
unmarried	47.5%	39.6%	$p < 0.05$
separated/divorced	6.8%	5.5%	
widows/ers	4.2%	7.4%	
Job occupation:			
housewife	14.8%	40.4%	$p < 0.01$
employed	26.9%	21.3%	
unemployed	13.5%	18.7%	
pensioner	13.5%	12.8%	
student	8.9%	6.8%	
unknown	16.6%	—	
Suicidal method:			
drug overdose	72.6%	59.1%	
cutting of veins	4.5%	31.5%	$p < 0.01$
caustic ingestion	6.6%	8.5%	
multiple methods	7.6%	—	
other methods	8.7%	0.9%	$p < 0.05$

X^2 (Yates' correction).

overdose (72.6 per cent in Padua and 59.1 per cent in ULSS No. 18), while the cutting of a vein was much more frequent in ULSS No. 18 (31.5 per cent of subjects) than in Padua (4.5 per cent). The next most common methods were ingestion of caustic substances (8.5 per cent in ULSS No. 18 and 6.6 per cent in Padua) and ingestion of foreign bodies (0.9 per cent in ULSS No. 18 and 2 per cent in Padua); 6.7 per cent of the Paduan subjects used other methods and 7.6 per cent made recourse to multiple methods.

A psychiatric diagnosis was formulated in 96 per cent of the ULSS No. 18 cases and 24.2 per cent of the Paduan cases. This comparison undoubtedly shows that the evaluation of suicidal drive induced very different clinical responses in the medical staff, since it does not seem realistic to believe that in one setting structured diagnoses were identified in almost all subjects, but in less than a quarter of the attempters in the other setting.

Statistical analysis showed that the incidence of attempted suicide was significantly higher in Padua. The difference in sex distribution was less marked than it was in the population of successful suicides, by reason of the far greater presence of women among the ULSS No. 18 attempted suicide population. The differences between the two populations with regard to marital and employment status were, however, more marked and highly significant.

Discussion and conclusions

Before proceeding to a discussion of the results obtained, some inevitable gaps in our work should be noted.

First of all, it should be noted that two different sources were used in the collection of data on suicidal behaviour (*carabinieri* and the registrar's office). This was, however, unavoidable in view of the fact that the source habitually considered most reliable (the local authority registers used in the collation of ISTAT's *Yearbook of Health Statistics*) proved entirely untrustworthy. In this context it should be said that examination of this latter register revealed that the forensic doctor had not formulated a diagnosis of suicide in numerous cases in which the circumstances of death lead naturally to this conclusion. The reasons for this behaviour are obscure, although the tendency of physicians in Italy to mask suicidal acts when possible has already been noted (De Leo *et al.* 1988). The Padua local authority register also tends to underestimate the real number of suicides, although apparently to a lesser extent.

It should also be noted that the total number of suicides (thirty-three) identified by ourselves in the ULSS No. 18 catchment area is rather small, and perhaps inadequate for the identification of salient characteristics of the behaviour. Moreover, there are deficiencies in the data from various other points of view: schooling level is unknown for most of the cases of suicide identified in the ULSS No. 18 catchment area, while the very high percentage (96 per cent) in which a psychiatric diagnosis was formulated seems to throw doubt on the overall reliability of this diagnosis. Furthermore, case histories were unavailable for suicides in both populations.

The most dramatic finding was that the incidence of suicide in the two territories considered was much higher than either the official national figure or that of the Veneto region—4.36 cases per year per 100 000 of population for the years 1974–83 (ISTAT, 1984). It is worth noting that our figures are almost 100 per cent higher than those registered by ISTAT. This is not the place for an evaluation of the possible reasons underlying this discrepancy. However, there is sufficient evidence to suppose that this understatement is a nationwide phenomenon.

The specific features of the social role of women in a rural environment probably explain the considerable difference between the distribution of suicides by sex. It should, in fact, be remembered that in the city of Padua many more women work outside the home, while housewives make up a larger proportion of the rural sample. It would appear that in the city the role of housewife (a major battle ground in the history of women's emancipation) is less acceptable than it is the outlaying areas, which may explain the higher percentage of housewives among the urban suicides.

Mean age is higher among the ULSS No. 18 population, but the most important finding concerns the distribution of cases among the age groups: 58 per cent of the ULSS No. 18 sample were aged over sixty, compared with only 34 per cent of suicides in Padua. Thus, it seems that the rural setting is less supportive of the elderly subject. The same consideration is valid for the higher percentage of unemployed committing suicide among the rural population (9 per cent as against 2 per cent).

The different distribution of subjects among the age groups probably also explains the differences found for other socio-demographic variables, such as the higher percentage of widows/ers in the ULSS No. 18 population and the lower percentage of married persons.

With regard to suicidal method, it is noteworthy that hanging was the most common method employed in the ULSS No. 18 sample. Defenestration was the second most frequent method in the Paduan population, while the second most frequent method in the ULSS No. 18 sample was drowning.

Attempted suicides were 30 per cent lower in the rural sample than in Padua. Females represented a higher proportion of the total in both samples, but most clearly so in the ULSS No. 18 sample. The mean age of suicide attempters in the ULSS No. 18 sample was appreciably higher than in the Paduan sample.

There were considerable differences between the two attempted suicide samples with regard to marital status. In the ULSS No. 18 sample the incidence of attempted suicide was highest amongst married people, while the unmarried were the most likely to attempt suicide in Padua.

One last difference in the socio-demographic characteristics of the two samples was that 40 per cent of the cases of attempted suicides in the ULSS No. 18 catchment area were by housewives, compared with only 15 per cent of the Paduan sample.

With regard to methods employed, an important difference was found in the incidence of vein cutting, which was very frequent in the ULSS No. 18 sample. It seems likely that this very dramatic method is perceived as likely to have a greater impact on the surrounding environment.

Thus, our analysis shows the existence of appreciable differences between the expression of self-destructive behaviours in the rural and urban settings. Unfortunately, the limits of our study prevent us from attaining a full understanding of the reasons underlying these differences. Nor can we exclude the possibility that the differences may, in some way, have been amplified by greater underestimation in the rural setting. However, it does seem possible to identify different patterns of suicidal behaviour in the two realities investigated: in the rural setting, suicide seemed to be less frequent and men were the main protagonists; while in Padua, both sexes committed suicide in almost equal proportions. Perhaps it would not be too incautious to deduce that the greater risk for women in the urban area is the failure to acquire an occupational position. In the rural setting, furthermore, the elderly seem more exposed to the risk of suicide than in the city, and the most common suicidal methods are more violent.

Attempted suicides are also less frequent in the rural zone than in Padua, where they are less common in the younger age groups and, unlike successful suicides, involve a large number of housewives. Lastly, the use of the more dramatic methods, such as cutting a vein, are more common in the rural setting.

One last and important consideration concerns the wide discrepancy found between official statistics and the data revealed by our survey: ISTAT reports suicide rates of about 5 per 100 000 for Padua and province, while the mean rate over a four-year period found by ourselves was 11 per 100 000. This can only be construed as a clear sign of a consistent underestimation of suicide.

References

Cecere, F. and Florenzano, F. 1984). 'Il suicidio in Italia', *G. Neuropsico-Farmacologia*, 6, 301–4.

De Leo, D., Banon, D. and Citron, P., *et al.* (1987). 'The guest for Reliable Epidemiological Data on Suicide: The Padua Sample', Paper presented at the 14th Congress of the IASP, San Francisco.

—— (1988). 'Il suicidio in Padova, 1986: Relazione presentata al I° Congresso Nazionale A.I.S.P.S.', Padova: Liviana Press.

Diekstra, R.F.W. (1985). 'Suicide and Suicide Attempts in the EEC: An Analysis of Trends, with Special Emphasis upon Trends Among the Young', *Suic Life Behav*, 15, 27–42.

Istituto Centrale di Statistica (ISTAT)(1980–5). *Annuari di Statistiche Sanitarie 1975–1980.* Roma: Istat.

Istituto Centrale di Statistica (1984). 'Dati Statistici sui Suicidi e Tentativi di Suicidio Anni 1974–1983', *Supplemento Bollettino Mensile di statistica*, 18, Roma: Istat.

Jacobson, L. and Renberg, E. (1985) 'Epidemiology of Suicide in a Swedish County (Vasterboten), 1961–1980', *Acta Psych Scand*, 74, 459–68.

WHO (1982). *Changing Patterns in Suicide Behaviour*, Copenhagen: Regional Office for Europe.

3

SUICIDAL BEHAVIOURS AND PSYCHIATRIC ILLNESS

Mortality and rate of suicide among first admission psychiatric patients[1]

ST. BLUMENTHAL, V. BELL, N.-U. NEUMANN,
R. SCHÜTTLER and R. VOGEL

Introduction

The majority of the studies dealing with the topic of suicide (Shneidman 1976; Shneidman and Farberow, 1961; Beck *et al.* 1974) are *ex post facto* investigations, i.e. the collection of relevant data from hospital records takes place after the fact, usually in an unsystematic manner. It is common knowledge that a retrospective approach is perhaps economical, but open to criticism of its methodology. When the topic of suicide is investigated in patients of a psychiatric hospital, more often than not the patients who are studied have already made a suicide attempt, have expressed suicidal tendencies, or are possible readmissions (Wolfersdorf *et al.* 1984; 1986). In this context, the following fact should be taken into consideration: the more distant the index suicide attempt, the greater the possibility that uncontrolled factors have had an influence on the completed suicide. Therefore, it would be wise to identify persons in danger of suicide as soon as possible.

The present study attempts to address this particular point of criticism. Most importantly, it is a prospective longitudinal study in which the data were systematically collected during and after the respective hospital stay. The data on patients who had committed suicide within the period before the five-year follow-up were used in the study. Also of importance is the fact that we studied only first admission psychiatric patients. This enabled us to limit the study to patients who were still in an early phase of the mental illness which afflicted them. The patient's first contact with institutional psychiatry was chosen as 'day 1' of a study period.

Method

The primary sample of this study consists of 258 first admission psychiatric patients of the Guenzburg Regional Hospital, who had been admitted in 1979. Concerning diagnoses, the sample consisted of patients with organic psychiatric illness (n = 21); schizophrenic psychoses (n = 33); depressive illness (n = 23); neurotic or psychosomatic illnesses, personality disorders and short-term emotional disorders (n = 81); and alcoholism and drug dependency (n = 100). In addition to the discharge interview/examination which took place in the clinic, we interviewed patients a second time after one year (one-year follow-up) and a final time after five years (five-year follow-up). In order to answer the questions posed in this study, we investigated how many of the original 258 patients committed suicide and how many died due to natural causes. A comparison of these two groups appeared interesting since recent research results indicate that former psychiatric patients have a higher mortality after discharge, not only due to unnatural causes (suicide) but also to natural (medical) causes (Winokur and Black, 1987). In a further control group, the suicide patients were matched with patients of the original sample according to the following traits: diagnosis, sex, age, and education. When possible, matching also included the additional criteria of marital status and occupational training.

The results given in this study originate from two general sources of data: the above-mentioned interview/examinations and the medical records of the patients in question. The interviews were carried out with the help of self-designed, structured questionnaires and standardised questionnaires. The psychopathological findings were determined with the PSE (Present State Examination, Wing *et al.* 1973). In the analysis of pre-hospital predictors, the following variables were taken into consideration: occupation (before and after first admission), job security, problems on the job, and an index of formal occupational integration. This index contains questions regarding actual time/days spent working, actual time/days spent *not* working, changes in qualifications, status of employment (i.e. civil servant, salaried, or hourly paid), and number of jobs. Further variables included motivation to work, contentment with work, plus a subjective judgement of the patient's achievement behaviour, and a prognosis index which was completed by the patient, the doctor, and a representative of the nursing staff. Furthermore, we also considered *clinical* variables, such as the discharge diagnosis, the psychopathological findings, and the duration of the entire hospital stay.

Results

During the five years after discharge, twelve patients (nine male; three female) committed suicide and twelve patients (eleven male; one female) died of natural causes (control group 1). Five patients of the suicide group were single, six were married, and one was divorced. The educational status in the majority of this group was 'Volksschulbidung', or primary/junior high school followed by vocational training. Of the two remaining patients, one completed 'Sonderschule' or a school for the mentally retarded, and another completed 'Realschule' or a junior high/senior school intended for intermediate-level business employees. Their age varied between twenty-two and forty-eight years, with an average of 34.3 years.

The diagnostic breakdown (ICD, 8th Edition) of the two samples at the five-year follow-up is shown in Tables 2 and 3).

It is evident that the diagnosis 303.2 (alcoholic addiction) is the diagnostic group with the highest risk of suicide, and natural death. These findings are at least partly explained by the fact that a high percentage (39 per cent) of the overall sample belongs to this diagnostic group.

A comparison between suicide and natural deaths shows an important difference in the period in which the patients died (Table 3). While only two patients from control group 1 had died before the one-year follow-up, whereas half the suicide group had already died. This shows clearly that potential suicide patients are particularly at risk in the first year after discharge.

The method in which patients committed suicide is documented in Table 4. A quarter of the patients chose death by hanging and another quarter by an intentional car accident. The methods used by the rest of the patients varied widely.

TABLE 1: Distribution of sex

	Suicide	*Natural death*
Male	9	11
Female	3	1
	12	12

TABLE 2: Distribution of discharge diagnoses at the five-year follow-up

Diagnosis ICD-8	*Suicide*		*Natural death*	
	n	%	*n*	%
291.2 Alcoholic hallucinosis	1	8.3	—	—
292.3 Psychosis associated with other and unspecified encephalitis	—	—	1	8.3
294.4 Psychosis associated with childbirth	1	8.3	—	—
295.2 Catatonic type of schizophrenia	1	8.3	—	—
295.3 Paranoid type of schizophrenia	2	16.6	—	—
296.0 Involutional melancholia	—	—	1	8.3
298.0 Reactive depressive psychosis	1	8.3	—	—
300.4 Depressive neurosis	1	8.3	—	—
303.0 Episodic excessive drinking	—	—	1	8.3
303.1 Habitual excessive drinking	—	—	2	16.6
303.2 Alcoholic addiction	4	33.3	7	58.3
307.0 Transient situational disturbances	1	8.3	—	—
Total	12	100.0	12	100.0

The causes of death in Control group 1 are given in Table 5. In control group 1 the patients who died from cancer predominated, with more than 40 per cent followed by a quarter who died from a poor general state of health (e.g. cardiovascular disease, alcohol-induced cardiomyopathy, etc.).

The primary goal of this study was to attempt to identify prehospital predictors of suicide. For this reason, we formed a second control group. Control group 2 consisted of twelve patients whose socio-demographic characteristics (diagnosis, sex, age, education) match those of the suicide cases.

The trait of occupation (before and after admission) is the first

TABLE 3: Distribution of the discharge diagnosis of (deaths) at the 1-year follow-up

Diagnosis	*Suicide*	*Natural death (Control Group 1)*
291.2 Alcoholic hallucinosis	1	—
292.3 Psychosis associated with other and unspecified encephalitis	—	1
295.3 Paranoid type of schizophrenia	1	—
298.0 Reactive depressive psychosis	1	—
303.2 Alcoholic addiction	3	1
Total	6	2

TABLE 4: Method of suicide and resulting numbers

Method	*Number of patients*
Hanging	3
Car accident	3
Inhalation of car exhaust fumes	1
Setting oneself on fire	1
Fall from a window	1
Drowning	1
Self-inflicted gunshot wound	1
Drug overdose (tablets)	1
Total	12

variable we chose to study (Table 6). In analysing these statistics, it is evident that a significantly higher number of the suicide patients were not in possession of a place of employment during their hospital stay compared with control groups 1 and 2.

The variable 'problems on the job' showed a significant difference between the suicide group and control group 1. There was, however, no difference between the suicide group and control group 2 (Table 7).

With respect to the variables 'motivation to work' and 'contentment with one's work', the suicide cases show a significant tendency which contrasts to the two control groups. The patients who had taken their lives had expressed a lower 'motivation to work' ($p = 0.07$) and less 'contentment with one's work' ($p = 0.09$) compared with the control groups. Variables which were not significantly different between groups included: 'subjective judgement of achievement behaviour', 'job security', 'prognosis of future occupational integration from the patient, the doctor, and a representative from the nursing staff', and the self-designed 'index of formal occupational integration'.

In observing the clinical variables, it is apparent that the

TABLE 5: Cause of natural death and resulting numbers

	Number of patients
1. Cancer	5
2. Poor general state of health	3
3. Cirrhosis of the liver	2
4. Cerebral abscess	1
5. Cardiac infarction	1
Total	12

TABLE 6: Occupation at the time of admission

	Suicide group	*Control group 1*	*Control group 2*	*Total*
In possession of a place of employment	7	12	11	30
Not in possession of a place of employment	5	—	1	6
Total	12	12	12	36

x^2 (S/I) = 5.0 p = 0.02
x^2 (S/II) = 3.5 p = 0.05.

TABLE 7: Problems in current/last job

	Suicide group	*Control group 1*	*Control group 2*	*Total*
Problems	6	1	6	13
No problems	6	11	6	23
Total	12	12	12	36

x^2 = 5.0 p = 0.02.

TABLE 8: Mean duration of hospital stay

Suicide group	*Control group 1*	*Control group 2*
days	*days*	*days*
67.0	79.3	88.7

TABLE 9: Frequency of pre-hospital symptoms

	Suicide group	*Control group 1*	*Control group 2*
1. Suicide attempt or thoughts	6	2	8
2. Isolation/desire for tranquility	6	—	4
3. Tiredness	1	—	2
4. Anxiety	3	1	4
5. Depressive mood	3	1	6
6. Hopelessness	3	—	2
7. Sleeplessness/sleep disturbances	3	—	4
8. Guilt feelings	3	—	1
9. Inner agitation/nervousness	4	1	4
10. Disruption in the family/Marital difficulties	6	6	7
11. Alcohol problems/addiction	8	10	8
Number of entries	47	21	50

duration of the hospital stay is different in each group (Table 8). Due to the small size of our sample, these differences do not reach significance.

The psychopathological finding (total PSE score) tends towards a significant difference ($p = 0.07$) between the suicide cases and control group 1, in which the former group expresses an elevated psychopathological symptomatology.

In order to examine the extent to which psychopathological symptoms stood out before the first hospital stay, we analysed the in-patient hospital records of the patients. A symptom list which we drew up for this purpose contained the following criteria shown in Table 9.

In this distribution of symptoms, a clear difference can be seen between the suicide cases and the patients who died of natural causes (control group 1) with respect to almost all symptoms (except for 'disruption of the family' and 'alcohol problems'); a comparison between suicide cases and control group 2, however, shows little difference.

Discussion and summary

To be able to prevent a suicide and to introduce individual therapeutic measures, it would be a great advantage for a doctor to know at the time of first admission which clues point towards a possible suicide or suicide attempt. The primary result of our data is the high suicide rate in patients with chronic alcohol abuse. This result coincides with other findings (Wolfersdorf *et al.* 1986) generally reported on suicide patients. In addition, our patients showed a particular vulnerability to suicide in the year following the (first) hospital stay.

In identifying predictors which have a connection to suicide, we found that suicidal patients, compared with the control groups, are more likely not to have a place of employment, and likewise, are less motivated to work and show less contentment with their work. Together, these results represent an initial stage or reason which justifies calling for further occupational rehabilitation measures after the patient's discharge from hospital.

The investigation of clinical variables showed a tendency towards elevated psychopathological findings in the suicide cases. Although the majority of these patients expressed such particular symptoms as a previous suicide attempt or suicidal thoughts, a tendency towards isolation, family disruption, and alcohol problems, this profile of symptoms did not differ in the matched control group.

It can, therefore, be concluded from the sample of our study that psychopathological symptoms cannot *alone* be seen as a predictor of suicide. Yet such clinicial variables *in combination with* occupational variables produce a general picture which, when pronounced, is associated with an increased probability of suicide.

Notes

1. The results of this study are part of a research project which is conducted at the Bezirkskrankenhaus Günsburg, Department of Psychiatry II of the University of Ulm (Prof. Dr. R. Schüttler, M.D.) and is sponsored by the German Research Association, Collaborative Research Program 129, Project A 1.

References

Beck, A.T., Schuyler, D. and Herman, J. (1974). 'Development of Suicidal Intent Scales', in A.T. Beck (ed.), *The Prediction of Suicide*, Maryland: Charles Press, 45–58.

Shneidman, E. (1976). 'An Overview of Suicide', *Psychiatr. Annals.* 6, 606–19.

—— and Farberow, N.L. (1961). 'Statistical Comparisons between Attempted and Committed Suicides', in: N.L. Farberow, E.S. Shneidman, (eds.), *The Cry for Help*, New York: McGraw-Hill, 19–47.

Wing, J.K., Cooper, J.E. and Sartorius, N. (1973). Present State Examination (PSE) 9, Fassung, Medical Research Council/Cambridge University Press.

Winokur, G. and Black, D.W. (1987). 'Psychiatric and Medical Diagnoses as Risk Factors for Mortality in Psychiatric Patients: A Case-Control Study', *Am. J. Psychiatry*, 2 (144), 208–11.

Wolfersdorf, M. (ed.) (1984). *Suicide psychiatrischer Patienten*, Weinsberg: Weissenhof-Verlag Dr. Jens Kunow.

——, Vogel, R., Hole, G., Dreher, D., Faulstich, H., Herr, W., Kirschmann, J., Metzger, R., Pröpper, D., Stoppa, H., Weiskittel, Ch. and Zlatnikova, J. (1986). 'Suicide psychisch Kranker in der psychiatrischen Klinik', in G. Laux and F. Reimer (eds.), *Klinische Psychiatrie. Band II*, Stuttgart: Hippokrates Verlag.

Schizophrenia and suicide in psychiatric in-patients

M. WOLFERSDORF, P. BARTH, B. STEINER, F. KELLER, R. VOGEL, G. HOLE and R. SCHÜTTLER

Introduction

In reports on suicide in the general population, schizophrenia is rarely mentioned; Robins *et al.* (1959) give a figure of 2 per cent, Dorpat and Riply (1960) of 11 per cent, Barraclough *et al.* (1974) of 3 per cent and Beskow (1979) of 6 per cent (males only) of suicides with the diagnosis of schizophrenia. In reports on attempted suicides it is even rarer: e.g. Feudell (1965) 4 per cent, Wedler 1984) 1.4 per cent, and Metzger and Schneider (1984) 2 per cent.

Suicide mortality among schizophrenics reaches 10 per cent in long-term follow-ups (Miles, 1977), and, according to Roy (1986), most of the schizophrenics (72 per cent) who commit suicide do so when not in in-patient psychiatric care.

According to our own studies, we find among schizophrenics in psychiatric hospitals approximately 12 per cent acutely and chronically suicidal patients (affective psychosis, ICD-9-296: 26 per cent). Hospital suicides are mainly schizophrenics: Wolfersdorf and Vogel (1987) found in a survey of nineteen hospital suicide studies 42 per cent with the diagnosis schizophrenia and 28 per cent with the diagnosis primary depression (endogenous and psychoreactive forms).

Thus it seems that outside the psychiatric hospital the group of schizophrenic patients is of little importance as far as suicide mortality is concerned (Kreitman, 1986), yet within the psychiatric hospital it is this group which accounts for most suicides.

It is, therefore, all the more striking that there have been few controlled studies of this group of patients which go beyond descriptions of warning signals. For instance, there are reports concerning the imminent suicide risk among patients with acoustic hallucinations urging them to commit suicide or concerning suicide proneness where paranoid delusions of persecution with threat to life appear (Jantz, 1951; Schüttler, 1987). Clinicians also know about suicide proneness in the so-called pharmacogenetic depression (Müller, 1982), although ideas about aetiology vary. Cohen *et al.* (1964) could not find any connection between neuroleptic therapy, depression and suicide among schizophrenics. Planansky and Johnston (1980) found depressive syndromes among schizophrenics just as often in the period prior to the administration of neuroleptics as in the period following it.

Apart from studies by Roy (1986), Breier and Astrachan (1984), Drake *et al.* (1984), and Salama (1987), there are few studies which compare schizophrenics who commit suicide while in in-patient care; there have never been any such comparative studies in German-speaking countries. This prompted us to carry out the research we are presenting here.

Sample, methods and questions

From the hospital suicide study carried out by the working group 'Suicide Proneness and the Psychiatric Hospital' (for more details, see Wolfersdorf and Vogel, 1987), we took 115 suicides (Hospital Suicides: HS) with the diagnosis ICD-9-295 schizophrenia and matched them for age ($\pm$ three years), sex and diagnosis with a group of in-patient schizophrenics who were still alive at the end of 1987 (Non-Hospital Suicides: NHS) and who had received in-patient treatment in the Weissenau County Psychiatric Hospital from 1986 to 1987. In both groups there were 72 (63 per cent) men and 43 (37 per cent) women. The average age in both groups was 40.5 years; the median was 39 years.

Two of the authors (MW, PB) collected the data. The statistical analyses were carried out at the computer centre of the University of Konstanz using the KOSTAS programme package (Nagl *et al.* 1987). Using the chi-square test, schizophrenics who committed suicide were compared to those who did not commit suicide while in in-patient care. Our aim was to find discriminating variables relevant to suicide. We collected the data using the Hospital-Suicide-Inquiry-Sheet which has been used for years by the working group 'Suicide Proneness and the Psychiatric Hospital' and which contains questions pertaining to the patient's life, to psychosocial variables and those relevant to the illness, the course of the illness and the symptoms, to in-patient stay and therapy as well as assessment of suicide proneness and any actual suicide attempt.

Selected results

Non-discriminating variables

In Table 1 we have drawn up a list of the variables which do not reveal significant differences between the groups. It is particularly striking that those variables which are mentioned in other studies as being significant, such as civil status, time out of gainful employment, developmental disorders in the early childhood, form of admission, number of in-patient stays as well as total duration of illness and ICD-9-295 subgroups, do not discriminate between groups. The assessment of suicide proneness made by the therapist on the patient's admission does not discriminate

TABLE 1: Schizophrenic hospital suicides (N = 115 HS) compared to schizophrenic in-patients without suicides (N = 115 NHS)

Civil status
Children
Composition of household
Schooling
Professional training, status
Time out of gainful employment
Employment corresponding to professional training
Pregnancy, birth
Type of difficulties
Type of early childhood developmental disorders
Unhappy childhood
Schizophrenia illness in family
Suicide/suicide attempt in the family
Admission
First in-patient treatment
Number of in-patient treatments
Total duration of illness (since first manifestation)
ICD-9-diagnosis 295 (subgroups)
Some of the symptoms on admission
Some of the reasons for admission
Period since last suicide attempt until index admission
Method used for last suicide attempt
Assessment of suicide proneness on admission
Special measures taken on admission because of suicide risk
Psycho-active medication
Other medication
Social therapy
Therapist in charge

Matched pairs: sex, age ± yrs, ICD-9: 925
Variables without significant difference (chi-square).

between groups either. Clinicians might expect that, compared to the patients who do not commit suicide, those who do are more often single, out of gainful employment, admitted against their will, and have repeatedly been in in-patient care, the total duration of their illness has been longer and they belong mainly to the ICD-9 subgroup 295.6 (schizophrenic residuum). Further, it is also thought that the patients who commit suicide are regarded already on admission as being suicidal and receive special therapeutic treatment and close observation because of suicide proneness.

Details of diagnoses and symptoms

Table 2 shows significant differences between HS and NHS groups on two variables relating to the course of the schizophrenic disorder. Schizophrenic hospital suicides, if they are patients who have been re-admitted, have a significantly longer penultimate in-patient stay and they are also more often re-admitted to hospital shortly after having last been discharged: 38 per cent of the patients who later commit suicide had a six-month or longer stay at their in-patient treatment; every fifth patient stayed for over a year; 59 per cent of hospital suicides had to be re-admitted after only six months; and every fourth (26 per cent) had to be re-admitted after four weeks.

Let us add that 48 percent of the suicides occur between the second and the fifth in-patient stay; a further 44 per cent of the suicides occur between the sixth and eight (inclusive) stay, and only 8 per cent of the schizophrenic patients (nine out of 117 cases) commit suicide during their very first in-patient stay. The high

TABLE 2: Course of schizophrenic disorder in hospital suicides (N = 115 HS) and non-hospital suicides (N = 115 NHS)

Variable	*Period (months)*	*Percentage of HS*	*NHS*	*Significance (chi-square)*
Length of last in-patient treatment before index admission	1	3	16	**
	1–2	36	51	
	3–5	23	19	
	6–12	18	10	
	12	20	4	
Period since last discharge until index admission	1	26	11	**
	1–2	19	13	
	3–5	14	9	
	6–12	20	26	
	12	21	41	

Matched pairs: sex, age ± 3 years, ICD-9: 295: significant differences.
** = p 0.01.

number of patients who are re-admitted after only a short time also explains why almost all the hospital suicides (92 per cent) were being treated in closed wards: 29 per cent in the emergency ward, 66 per cent in the medium-term ward, and 5 per cent in the long-term ward.

The prognosis which the therapists had made concerning the expected total course of the illness for the schizophrenic patients who later committed suicide was highly significantly bad ($p \leqslant 0.01$): hospital suicides; continuously or periodically bad with a tendency to worsen, 76 per cent as opposed to 56 per cent for the non-hospital suicides: tendency to improve; 6 per cent for the hospital suicides as opposed to 27 per cent for the non-hospital suicides. Again concerning the therapy results in the index treatment, there were highly significant differences ($p \leqslant 0.01$), the hospital suicides having a larger proportion of worsening and only a small proportion of improvements: worsening among hospital suicides, 22 per cent as opposed to 2 per cent among the non-hospital suicides; 44 per cent unchanged as against 26 per cent; improved and very much improved 34 per cent as opposed to 73 per cent.

Concerning symptoms (Table 3), it is striking that on admission the schizophrenic patients without hospital suicide are significantly more likely to have paranoid delusions of persecution and poisoning, have more often a secondary diagnosis of alcohol and drug abuse and, on the whole, suffer more often from visual and acoustic hallucinations (except for those imperative voices urging towards suicide which do not discriminate the groups). Patients in either group have just as many symptoms of depression, anxiety, inner restlessness, or psychomotoric inhibition; in other words, they present a clinical picture of anxiety-depression in the widest sense.

TABLE 3: Symptoms on admission, schizophrenic hospital suicides (N = 115 HS) compared to schizophrenic inpatients without suicide (N = 115 NHS)

Symptoms	*No (%) of* *HS*	*NHS*	*Significance (chi-square)*
Hallucinations other than imperative voices urging suicide	30	56	**
Paranoid ideas of persecution, poisoning	29	66	**
Alcohol and/or drug abuse	6	23	**

Matched pairs: sex, age ± 3 yrs, ICD-9: 295: significant differences.
** = $p < 0.01$.

Details of the assessment of suicide proneness

As we have shown above, the therapist's assessment of suicide proneness on admission does not discriminate between the groups. Approximately the same number of patients in either group is considered to be non-suicidal on admission. In either group there is also about the same number of patients with actual plans for, and intentions of, committing suicide, although there is a slightly higher percentage of patients in the suicide group who no longer wish to live and have concrete suicide thoughts, and a higher percentage of patients in the non-suicide group whom the therapists suspect of being suicidal. Consequently, measures are taken as often for one group as for the other to prevent suicide, such as placing the patients in closed wards, sedating them, and observing them continuously. The patients who later commit suicide, however, have significantly more often attempted to commit suicide either right up to the time of their index admission or during in-patient care. Suicide proneness in the widest sense is also more frequently ($p = 0.05$) the reason for admission among the patients who later commit suicide (Table 4).

Details of therapy

The main differences between the groups in respect of therapy are summed up in Table 5. Patients who later commit suicide are more frequently taking low-potent neuroleptics at the time they commit suicide and have more frequently had electric convulsive therapy in their case history. They have significantly less often had depot neuroleptics or psychotherapy based on a particular theory (Table 5). The patients who later commit suicide have to bear significantly more frequently (also in about one third of the cases) a change of therapist or treatment (especially of psycho-active drug therapy) or ward during the three months before suicide. On the other hand both groups are administered psycho-active medi-

TABLE 4: Suicidal behaviour prior to suicide, schizophrenic hospital suicides (N = 115 HS) versus schizophrenic in-patients without suicide (N = 115 NHS)

Behaviour	*No (%) of* *HS*	*NHS*	*Significance (chi-square)*
Suicide attempts priot to index admission	55	17	**
Suicide attempt during index treatment	20	3	**
Suicidality as a reason for hospital admission	35	17	*

Matched pairs: sex, age ± 3 years, ICD-9: 295: significant differences.
* = $p < 0.05$, ** = $p < 0.01$.

TABLE 5: Schizophrenic hospital suicides (N = 115 HS) compared with schizophrenic in-patients without suicide (N = 115 NHS), therapy: significant differences

Variable	*No (%) of* *HS*	*NHS*	*Significance (chi-square)*
Neuroleptics—low-potent medication	25	9	**
—high-potent medication	38	56	
—both	37	36	
Depot neuroleptics	54	82	**
Tranquilisers	23	14	
Hypnotics	19	4	
Previous ECT	30	10	**
Psychotherapy	20	94	**

** = $p < 0.01$.

TABLE 6: Changes in treatment strategies in the last three months before suicide in the hospital suicide group compared with in-patient treatment period of the non-suicide group

Variable	*No (%) of* *HS*	*NHS*	*Significance (chi-square)*
Change of therapist	37	4	**
Change of treatment	43	12	**
Change of ward	25	8	**

Schizophrenic hospital suicides (N = 115 HS) and schizophrenic non-hospital suicides (N = 115 NHS). Matched pairs: sex, age ± 3 years, ICD-9: 295: significant differences.
** = $p < 0.01$.

cation just as often; the same applies for anti-depressants and neuroleptics. There are no differences either concerning the prescription of tranquillisers, hypnotics, or social therapy.

Discussion

In this study we have attempted to find variables which discriminated between schizophrenics who commit suicide in hospital and those who do not commit suicide either in hospital or during the year following their in-patient stay. Relevant publications contain very few results: to date there has been nothing on the subject in German-speaking countries.

If we are to sum up the results of our study, we can describe the typical schizophrenic hospital suicide patient as follows: he is usually a youngish man, belonging mostly to the ICD-9 subgroups 295.3, 295.6 and 295.7 (without this being, however, a discriminating factor); he has been admitted to psychiatric hospital often and has, in particular, had long in-patient treatment; there is usually only a short interval between his last discharge from hospital and his index admission. Previous long in-patient stays and short periods outside hospital go along with bad prognosis concerning the further course of the illness and unsatisfactory therapy results during current in-patient treatment. As far as pharmacology is concerned, this patient has usually received subduing low-potent neuroleptics and, less often, in spite of repeated admissions and short-term re-admission, depot neuroleptics; he has seldom received psychotherapy based on a particular theory but has often been given electric convulsive therapy at some time in his history. Suicide proneness was obvious as much from the patient's history of suicide attempts as from the course of his current in-patient stay, although, on admission, suicides do not differ from non-suicides. On the whole, this describes a patient who, on the one hand, shows the traits of a long-term patient and, on the other, seems, time after time, to be a patient who can be discharged and is capable of rehabilitation (Leff and Wing, 1971; Stephens, 1978; Leff *et al.* 1984; Mundt, 1984, 1987; Gestrich, 1987).

At the time of admission the psychopathology does not seem particularly striking. Although a quarter of the hospital suicides show symptoms of depression and anxiety, withdrawal and psychomotoric inhibition, which corresponds to the number of patients under anti-depressant medication, this still does not discriminate between them and non-suicides. Hospital suicides have even significantly fewer hallucinations and delusions of reference. The number of imperative voices urging to suicide ranges between 3 per cent and 4 per cent, and is not discriminating. This confirms what Jantz stated as early as 1951: 'It is not true either when it is claimed that a schizophrenic commits suicide as a result of delusion, hallucinations or loss of relation to reality'. Imperative voices urging to suicide mean that there is a high suicide risk in each case, although on the whole they are seldom the cause of actual suicide; this can also be found in Breier and Astrachan (1984), Drake *et al.* (1984), and Roy (1986). Waxberg (1956), Simko (1983), and Quindt (1987) interpreted paranoid delusions of reference, such as feelings of being persecuted or poisoned, as projective defence mechanisms against depression and suicide proneness, which might explain their high occurrence among non-hospital suicides (NHS 66 per cent) as opposed to their rare occurrence among suicides. Our own results agree, by and large, with those of Drake *et al.* (1984), although they had more patients

TABLE 7: Suicides during the first six months of index in-patient treatment according to diagnosis

Month	*Affective Dis. (N = 33) (ICD-9: 296: without mania)* N	%	*Schizophrenia (N = 107) (ICD-9: 295)* N	%
First	12	36	12	11
Second	4	12	13	12
Third	3	9	9	8
Fourth	3	9	1	1
Fifth	–	–	7	7
Sixth	–	–	7	7
⩾Seventh	11	33	58	54

living alone, with depressive moods and suicidal thoughts, than we did.

This means that the aspects of the course of the patient's illness are more important, especially as far as the schizophrenic suicide is concerned, than actual psychopathology (Retterstol, 1987). This idea is reinforced by the fact that among schizophrenic hospital suicides the reasons for the suicidal act are psychoreactive: in 28 per cent of cases they concern relational problems within and beyond the ward as well as loneliness, and in 59 per cent of cases they concern the illness.

TABLE 8: Some important variables with significant difference ($p = < 0.01$)(chi-square), schizophrenic hospital suicides (N = 115 HS) compared with schizophrenic in-patients without suicide (N = 115 NHS)

Length of last in-patient treatment before index admission	HS > NHS
Period since last discharge until index admission	HS > NHS
Poorer course of illness	HS > NHS
Prognosis of assessment of poorer results during index treatment	HS > NHS
Paranoid ideas of persecution, poisoning	NHS > HS
Hallucinations (without imperative voices urging to suicide)	NHS > HS
Alcohol and/or drug abuse	NHS > HS
Suicide attempts before index admission	HS > NHS
Suicide attempts during index treatment	HS > NHS
Neuroleptic medication low-potent	HS > NHS
Depot neuroleptics	NHS > HS
Previous ECT	HS > NHS

The schizophrenic hospital suicide is a patient with a long illness and a first suicide peak during the first six months of in-patient care (Table 7); (on the other hand, patients with affective psychoses show a distinct suicide peak as early as in the first four weeks); the schizophrenic hospital suicides, which happen later, occur during the second year of in-patient care, the rest are divided across the five following years of in-patient care. In this period, it seems that re-admission shortly after an in-patient stay particularly promotes suicide. Retterstol (1987) has also given more importance to the course of the illness. This is striking if we have a look at the summary on Table 8.

References

Barraclough, B., Bunch, J., Nelson, B. and Sainsbury, P. (1974). 'A Hundred Cases of Suicide: Clinical Aspects', *Brit. J. Psychiat.* 125, 355–73.

Beskow, J. (1979). Suicide and Mental Disorder in Swedish Men', *Acta Psychiatr. Scand.* (*Suppl.*), 277, 5–128.

Breier, A. and Astrachan, B.M. 1984). 'Characterization of Schizophrenic Patients who Commit Suicide', *Am. J. Psychiatry*, 141, 206–9.

Cohen, S., Leonard, C.V., Farberow, N.L. and Shneidman, E.S. (1964). 'Tranquilizers and Suicide in the Schizophrenic Patient', *Arch Gen Psychiat.*, 11, 312–21.

Dorpat, Th.L., Ripley, H.S. (1960). 'A Study of Suicide in the Seattle Area', *Compreh. Psychiat.*, 1, 349–59.

Drake, R.E., Gates, Ch., Cotton, P.G. and Whitaker, A. (1984). 'Suicide among Schizophrenics: Who is at Risk?', *The Journal of Nervous and Mental Disease*, 172, 613–17.

Feudell, P. (1965). 'Epikrise zu 700 Selbstmordversuchen', in Ch. Zwingmann (ed.) *Selbstvernichtung*, Akademische Verlagsgesellschaft Frankfurt/Main, 35–46.

Gestrich, J. (1987). 'Über den Umgang mit suizidalen schizophrenen Patienten', in M. Wolfersdorf and R. Vogel (eds.) *Suizidalität bei stationären psychiatrischen Patienten*, Weinsberg: Weissenhof-Verlag Dr Jens Kunow, 147–59.

Jantz, H. (1951). 'Schizophrenie und Selbstmord', *Nervenarzt*, 2, 126–33.

Kreitman, N. (1986). 'Die Epidemiologie des Suizids und Parasuizids', in K.P. Kisker, H. Lauter, J.E. Meyer, C. Müller and E. Strömgen (eds.) *Psychiatrie der Gegenwart*, 2, Krisenintervention—Suizid—Konsiliarpsychiatrie, Springer Verlag, 87–106.

Leff, J., Knipers, L., Berkowitz, R., Eberlein-Fries, R. and Sturgeon, D. (1984). 'Psychosocial Relevance and Benefit of Neuroleptic Maintenance: Experience in the United Kingdom', *J. Clin. Psychiatry*, (Sec 2), 45, 43–49.

—— and Wing, J.K. (1971). 'Trial of Maintenance Therapy in Schizophrenia', *Br. Med. J.*, 111, 599–604.

Metzger, R. and Schneider, J. (1984). *Suizidversuche im Raum Ravensbrug. Eine sozialpsychiatrische Studie*, Weinsberg: Weissenhof-Verlag Dr Jens Kunow.

Miles, C. (1977). 'Conditions Predisposing to Suicide: A Review', *J. Nerv. Men. Dis.*, 164, 231–46.

Müller, P. (1982). *Zur Rezidivprophylaxe schizophrener Psychosen*, Stuttgart: Enke-Verlag.

Mundt, Ch. (1984). 'Suizide schizophrener Patienten. Überlegungen zur Genese und Prävention anhand einiger Fallbeispiele', *Psychother. med. Psychol.*, 34, 193–7.

—— (1987). 'Spezifische und unspezifische Risikofaktoren für Suizide Schizophrener und der therapeutische und präventive Umgang mit ihnen', in M. Wolfersdorf and R. Vogel (eds.), *Suizidalität bei stationären psychiatrischen Patienten*, Weinsberg: Weissenhof-Verlag Dr Jens Kunow, 107–30.

Nagl, W., Walter, H.-G. and Staud, J.L. (1987) (eds), *Statistische Verfahren der empirischen Sozialforschung in einem Programmpaket. Das Konstanzer Statistische Analysesystem KOSTAS*, Forschungsberichte 47/1 und 2, Universität Konstanz.

Planansky, K. and Johnston, R. (1980). 'Psychotropic Drugs and Depressive Syndrome in Schizophrenia', *Psychiatric Quarterly*, 52, 214–21.

Quint, H. (1987). 'Psychodynamische Aspekte paranoider Reaktionen und Entwicklungen', in H.M. Olbrich (ed.), *Halluzinationen und Wahn*, Springer-Verlag, 140–9.

Retterstöl, N. (1987). 'Schizophrenie—Verlauf und Prognose', in K.P. Kisker, H. Lauter, J.-E. Meyer, *et al.* (eds.), *Psychiatrie der Gegenwart, 4, Schizophrenien*, Springer-Verlag, 71–115.

Robins, E., Gassner, S., Kayes, J. *et al.* (1959). 'The Communication of Suicidal Intent: A Study of 134 Consecutive Cases of Successful Suicide', *Am. J. Psychiatry*, 115, 724–33.

Roy, A. (1986). 'Suicide in schizophrenia', in A. Roy (ed.), *Suicide*, Baltimore: Williams & Wilkins, 97–112.

Salama, A.A. (1987). Depression and Suicide in Schizophrenic Patients', Paper presented at the Conference of the American Association of Suicidology (AAS) and the International Association for Suicide Prevention (IASP), San Francisco, 25–30 May, *Conference Proceedings*, Denver: AAS Denver, 375–7.

Schüttler, R. (1987). 'Suizidalität im Verlauf schizophrener Psychosen', in M. Wolfersdorf and R. Vogel (eds.), *Suizidalität bei stationären psychiatrischen Patienten*, Weinsberg: Weissenhof-Verlag, Dr Jens Kunow, 131–46.

Simko, A. (1983). 'Zur Psychopathologie der Schuldwahndepressionen', in G. Gross and R. Schüttler (eds.), *Empirische Forschung in der Psychiatrie*, Stuttgart: Schattauer Verlag, 129–38.

Stephens, J.H. (1978). 'Long-term Prognosis and Follow-up in Schizophrenia', *Schizophrenia Bull.*, 4, 25–37.

Waxberg, J.D. (1956). 'Study of Attempted Suicides in Psychotic Patients: A Dynamic Concept', *Psychiat. Quart.*, 33, 464–70.

Wedler, H. (1984). *Der Suizidpatient im Allgemeinkrankenhaus*, Stuttgart: Enke Verlag.

Wolfersdorf, M. and Vogel, R. (eds.)(1987a). *Suizidalität bei stationären psychiatrischen Patienten. Tagungsprotokolle der Arbeitsgemeinschaft 'Suizidalität und psychiatrisches Krankenhaus' und weitere Beiträge*, Weinsberg: Weissenhof-Verlag Dr Jens Kunow.

—— (1987b). 'Types of Hospital Suicide and Depression', *Crisis*, 8, 37–48.

Suicidal behaviour in schizophrenic patients: a follow-up investigation

A. ROHDE, A. MARNEROS and A. DEISTER

Introduction

It is generally agreed that amongst psychotic (particularly schizophrenic) patients there is a high risk of suicide and attempted suicide (Allebeck and Wistedt, 1986; Black *et al.* 1985; Drake *et al.* 1984, 1985, 1986; Pickar *et al.* 1986; Roy, 1985). The aims of the present study are, therefore, to investigate (*a*) how often suicidal behaviour occurs during the long-term course of schizophrenia; (*b*) whether there are certain schizophrenic patients in whom the risk of suicidal behaviour is higher than in others; (*c*) whether there is a point in the course of the illness when the risk is especially high; or (*d*) whether there are particular circumstances which seem to 'produce' or 'support' suicidal behaviour. To answer these questions we investigated suicidal behaviour during the course of schizophrenia in ninety-seven patients.

Materials and methods

The ninety-seven schizophrenic patients referred to in this chapter were investigated as part of the Cologne study on the long-term course and outcome of psychoses (Marneros *et al.* 1986a,b,c, 1989a,b; Steinmeyer *et al.* 1989). They were categorised as schizophrenic from a total of 205 patients interviewed by us after a mean duration of illness of 19.6 years (for instruments of the follow-up investigation see Table 1). The criteria given in Marneros *et al.* (1986a, 1988a) were used. Schizophrenia is defined as a mental disorder with schizophrenic symptomatology according to DSM-III (with slight modifications, Marneros *et al.* 1986a, 1988a), but with no melancholic or manic symptomatology during

TABLE 1: Instruments of evaluation

Instruments of follow-up investigation
1. PSE = Present State Examination (Wing *et al.* 1982)
2. Modified version of PSE for follow-up (follow-up PSE)
3. Course and outcome protocol:
(*a*) DAS = Disability Assessment Schedule (WHO 1978, 1986)(*)
(*b*) FU-HSD = Follow-up history and Socio-demographic Description Schedule (WHO)(**)
(*c*) DHSD = Past history and Socio-demographic Description Schedule (WHO)(**)
(*d*) PIRS = Psychological Impairment Rating Schedule (WHO, 1986)(*)
(*e*) GAS = Global Assessment Scale (Spitzer *et al.* 1976)
(*f*) Own completions, i.e. socio-demographic data, therapy, etc.
4. Case record evaluation protocol
(*a*) Socio-demographic data
(*b*) Family history
(*c*) Broken home
(*d*) Life events
(*e*) History of illness
(*f*) Psychopathological symptoms (AMDP oriented)
(*g*) Somatic findings
(*h*) Treatment
(*i*) Course and outcome of episode

(*) Schubarth *et al.* (1986)
(**) WHO (1979a)

the whole course of the illness. Some features of the population in the study are shown in Table 2.

We investigated suicidal behaviour in the whole population in the study as well as in every single hospitalisation amongst the ninety-seven patients (402 hospitalisations altogether; for the eighteen permanently hospitalised patients only hospitalisations before this event were included). 'Suicidal behaviour' in this chapter means admission to a psychiatric hospital because of attempted suicide or suicidal intentions, or suicidal symptoms during hospitalisation. As far as possible we also recorded suicidal behaviour between hospitalisations and before first admission. We investigated suicidal intentions separately from attempted suicide.

Results

Suicidal behaviour in each patient

Of the schizophrenic patients investigated, 54 per cent showed suicidal symptomtology (suicidal intentions or attempted suicide) at least once during the course of their illness; 19 per cent of the

TABLE 2: Features of study population

Cologne study—schizophrenia (N = 97)				
Sex	female	(N = 42)	43%	ratio 0.76:1
	male	(N = 55)	57%	
Age at onset (years)				Median = 25.0
				Mean = 29.89
				s.d. = 11.60
				Min. = 15.00
				Max. = 64.00
Age at end of follow-up period (years)				Median = 49.00
				Mean = 49.46
				s.d. = 13.85
				Min. = 27.00
				Max. = 84.00
Duration of follow-up period (years)				Median = 18.00
				Mean = 19.58
				s.d. = 8.80
				Min. = 10.00
				Max. = 39.00
Patients personally interviewed				100%
Place of interview				
—Patients visited us				24%
—Patients were visited at home				55%
—Psychiatric hospital/care unit				22%
Patients' relatives or relevant familiar persons interviewed additionally				36%

patients displayed suicidal symptoms at least twice; 37 per cent of the investigated sample attempted suicide at least once during the course of the illness. Altogether, then, more than two-thirds of the patients with suicidal symptomatology had, in fact, attempted suicide.

No significant differences between suicidal and non-suicidal schizophrenic patients were found regarding age or marital status at onset or at follow-up, education and vocational training, the parents' social class, the patient's social class at onset or at the end of the observation time, the highest achieved social class, downward social mobility, the presence of residuum at follow-up, the severity of residuum, the number of admissions, the mean duration of intervals between hospitalisations, 'broken home' situation before the age of sixteen, or psychiatric illnesses or suicide in the family. The only relevant difference between suicidal and non-suicidal patients was the sex of the patients: female schizophrenic patients were found to display suicidal

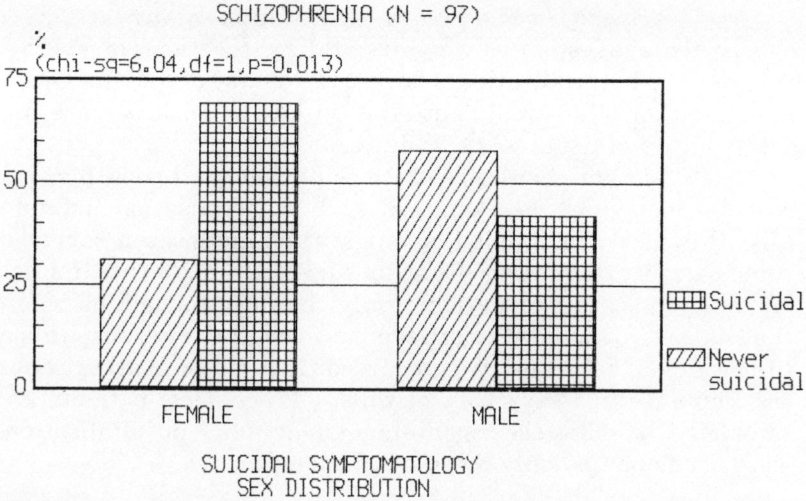

Figure 1: Suicidal symptomatology

symptomatology significantly more frequently than male schizophrenic patients (69 per cent compared with 42 per cent, p = 0.013; see also Fig. 1). Females were also found to attempt suicide significantly more often than males (50 per cent compared with 29 per cent, p = 0.024, Fig. 2).

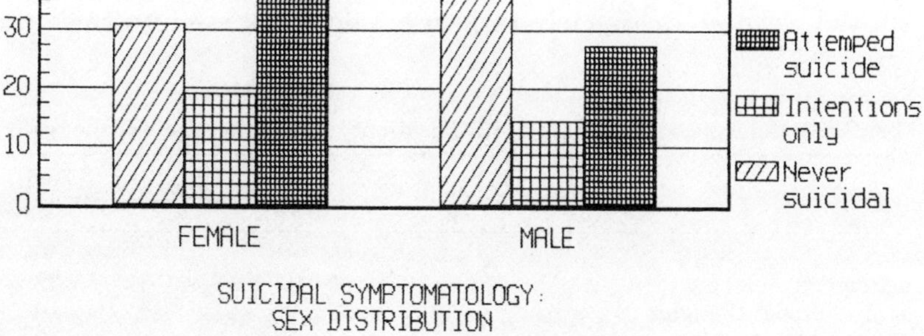

Figure 2: Suicidal symptomatology and behaviour.

Suicidal behaviour in 402 hospitalisations

The patients investigated were hospitalised 4.29 times on average (range: 1–20 hospitalisations) during the course of the illness, and had in-patient-like treatments (i.e. intensive medical care and interruption of usual work or duties).

To find out whether there are specific factors correlating with suicidal behaviour we examined each hospitalisation individually. Previously mentioned, amongst the ninety-seven schizophrenic patients there were 402 hospitalisations altogether (for permanently hospitalised patients only the hospitalisations before that time were included). For seventy-one of these 402 hospitalisations suicidal behaviour was recorded (18 per cent of all episodes, see Table 3). In forty-seven of them (12 per cent) patients had attempted suicide; the remaining twenty-four hospitalisations were accompanied only by suicidal thoughts.

Non-symptomatological factors at the time of every hospitalisation

We tried to discover whether there were some non-symptomatological factors (for instance, age at the time of hospitalisation, marital status, occupation, or precipitating events) which correlate with suicidal symptoms in relapses of illness. As shown in Table 4, the age at the time of hospitalisation did not differ significantly between suicidal and non-suicidal schizophrenic relapses. In 79 per cent of the suicidal and 76 per cent of the non-suicidal episodes the patients were below forty years of age. There was also no difference regarding marital status at the time of hospitalisation (60 per cent single, 30 per cent married, 10 per cent divorced or widowed). Another of the factors investigated was the employment situation of the patient at the time of hospitalisation. We found no significant differences between the suicidal and non-suicidal group of hospitalisations. Being unemployed, retired, or in early retirement does not seem to raise the suicidal risk.

TABLE 3: Schizophrenia (single hospitalisations): suicidal symptomatology

	Suicidal *(N = 71)*	*Total* *(N = 402)*
	%	%
Attempted suicide	*66*	12
Only suicidal thoughts	*34*	6
No suicidal symptomatology	—	82

TABLE 4: Schizophrenia (single hospitalisations) non-symptomatological factors at time of episode

	No suicidal symptoms (N = 331)	*Suicidal (N = 71)*	*Total (N = 402)*	*p*
	%	%	%	
Age at time of episode:				ns
Up to 40 years	76	*79*	77	
41–60 years	20	*20*	20	
61 years and older	4	*1*	4	
Occupational state at time of episode:				ns
Employed	40	*42*	41	
Unemployed	22	*17*	21	
Housewife	15	*20*	16	
Retired	1	*1*	1	
Retired early (psychiatric reason)	22	*20*	21	
Life event before episode:				0.04
Life event present	9	*18*	11	
No life event	91	*82*	89	

Eighteen per cent of the suicidal hospitalisations were preceded by a stressful life event. This is twice as high as the percentage in the non-suicidal group. But it has to be considered that in only 11 per cent of the total hospitalisations were there precipitating factors (Table 4).

Symptomatological factors at the time of hospitalisation
We also investigated whether there were certain psychopathological constellations which correlate with suicidal behaviour in connection with hospitalisation. For instance, we evaluated whether there was a residual state at the time of any single hospitalisation. There were four patients in our schizophrenic population in whom the time of the beginning of the residuum was unknown and their hospitalisations were excluded. We compared first admissions to hospital, who by definition had no residual symptomatology with hospitalisations later in the course of the illness with or without residual psychopathology. We found a significant difference in suicidal behaviour ($p = 0.0014$), with most frequent suicidality amongst first admissions (42 per cent). On comparing only hospitalisations with and without residual symptomatology later in the course of the illness no significant difference was found (Table 5). This means that neither the

TABLE 5: Schizophrenia (single hospitalisations) episodes with and without residual symptoms

Residual symptoms	*No suicidal symptoms (N = 320)*	*Suicidal (N = 67)*	*Total (N = 387)*	*p*
	%			
First episode	21	42	25	
Later episode without residuum	5	5	5	
Later eipsode with residuum	74	54	71	

presence nor the absence of residual symptoms plays a role, but what it does mean is whether it is the first hospitalisation or in-patient like treatment for a patient, or whether it is later in the course of the illness which is important.

We also investigated the role of different psychopathological symptoms. Suicidal behaviour was recorded in 33 per cent of the hospitalisations accompanied by depressive symptoms (other than a melancholic symptom-constellation), nearly twice the rate for all hospitalisations. But suicidality was also present in 15 per cent of the hospitalisations with manifold symptoms.

Regarding productive psychotic symptomatology we found no single symptom which correlated with a significant difference in suicidality (Table 6). The presence of incoherence did not differentiate between the groups. Comparing the hospitalisations with positive, negative, and positive–negative mixed episodes according to Andreasen and Olsen (1982), we found that positive–negative mixed episodes had the highest percentage of suicidal beha-

TABLE 6: Schizophrenia (single hospitalisation): psychopathology

	No suicidal symptoms (N = 331)	*Suicidal (N = 71)*	*Total (N = 402)*	*p*
	%	%	%	
Hallucinations (total)	19	27	20	ns
Acoustic hallucinations	18	24	19	ns
Delusions (total)	45	48	46	ns
Paranoid–hallucinatory symptomatology	18	28	20	ns
First-rank symptoms	15	17	15	ns
Incoherence	18	20	18	ns

chi-square-test: ** = $p < 0.01$, * = $p < 0.05$, ns = not significant

TABLE 7: Schizophrenia (single hospitalisations): suicidal symptomatology in different types of episode

		Suicidal
Positive symptoms	(N = 181)	16%
Negative symptoms	(N = 105)	18%
Positive–negative mixed symptoms	(N = 61)	25%
Missing informations	(N = 55)	16%

viour (Table 7). However, the differences were not statistically significant.

Methods of attempted suicide

Table 8 shows of attempted suicide in forty-five episodes the most common method was intoxication with pills (73 per cent). So-called hard methods were used in only 22 per cent of cases (cutting, 15 per cent; hanging, 7 per cent).

Suicidal behaviour in intervals and before first admission

In addition to suicidal symptomatology in connection with hospitalisations, we recorded suicidal behaviour in 8.2 per cent of all intervals between two admissions or hospitalisation-like treatment. This means that patients without acute psychotic symptomatology had serious suicidal thoughts or had even attempted suicide and were not treated or transferred to a hospital. It seems of particular importance to us that fourteen of the ninety-seven patients had already displayed suicidal behaviour before the first observed clinical manifestation of schizophrenia.

Conclusions

Suicidal symptomatology was investigated in ninety-seven

TABLE 8: Schizophrenia (single hospitalisations); methods of attempted suicide

	Attempted suicide (N = 45)
Drug intoxication	73%
Cutting artery	13%
Hanging	7%
Poisoning	2%
Cutting throat	2%

schizophrenic patients during the long-term course of their illness. We found that more than half of the patients displayed suicidal behaviour at least once during course and that half of these patients attempted suicide. Female schizophrenic patients displayed suicidal symptomatology more frequently than male schizophrenic patients; they also attempted suicide more frequently.

Investigating the seventy-one hospitalisations accompanied by suicidal symptoms (of 402 total admissions), hospitalisations with or without suicidal behaviour did not differ regarding age, marital status, or employment situation of the patient at the time of hospitalisation. No single psychopathological symptom differentiated suicidal and non-suicidal hospitalisations. Regarding positive and negative symptoms, hospitalisations with positive–negative mixed episodes had the highest rate of suicidal behaviour, but this was not statistically significant. In hospitalisations accompanied by depressive symptoms, suicidal symptoms were present in one-third of the cases, but also in 15 per cent of admissions with manifold symptoms besides the schizophrenic picture.

Precipitating factors were found significantly more frequently before admissions accompanied by suicidal symptomatology, but the frequency was not, in fact, high. The presence of residual symptomatology does not seem to change the risk of suicidal behaviour. Patients hospitalised later in the course of the illness are less at risk than first admissions. The most common method of attempted suicide was intoxication with pills; only seldom were 'hard' methods recorded.

References

Allebeck, P. and Wistedt, B. (1986). 'Mortality in Schizophrenia', *Archives of General Psychiatry*, 43, 650–3.

Andreasen, N.C. and Olsen, S. (1982). 'Negative vs Positive Schizophrenia: Definition and Validation', *Archives of General Psychiatry*, 39, 789–94.

Black, D.W., Winokur, G. and Warrack, G. (1985). 'Suicide in Schizophrenia: The Iowa Record Linkage Study', *Journal of Clinical Psychiatry*, 46, 14–17.

Drake, R.E., Gates, C. and Cotton, P.G. (1986). 'Suicide among Schizophrenics: A Comparison of Attempters and Completed Suicides', *British Journal of Psychiatry*, 149, 784–7.

—— and Whitacker, A. (1984). 'Suicide among Schizophrenics', *Journal of Nervous and Mental Disease*, 172, 613–17.

—— (1985). 'Suicide among Schizophrenics: A Review', *Comprehensive Psychiatry*, 26, 90–9.

Marneros, A., Deister, A. and Rohde, A. (1986a). 'The Cologne Study on Schizoaffective Disorders and Schizophrenia Suspects', in A. Marneros and M.T. Tsuang (eds.), *Schizoaffective Psychoses*, Springer.

Marneros, A., Rohde, A. and Deister, A. (1986b). 'Features of Schizoaffective Disorders: The "Cases-in-between"', in A. Marneros and M.T. Tsuang (eds.), *Schizoaffective Psychoses*, Springer.

—— and Risse, A. (1986c). 'Schizoaffective Disorders: The Prognostic Value of the Affective Component', in A. Marneros and M.T. Tsuang (eds.), *Schizoaffective Psychoses*, Springer.

Marneros, A., Deister, A., Rohde, A., Jünemann, H. and Fimmers, R. (1988a). 'Long-term Course of Schizoaffective Disorders: Definitions, Methods, Frequency of Episodes and Cycles', *European Archives of Psychiatry and Neurological Sciences*, 237, 264–75.

Marneros, A., Deister, A., Rohde, A., Steinmeyer, E.M. and Jünemann, H. (1989a). 'Long-term Outcome of Schizoaffective and Schizophrenic Disorders: A Comparative Study: Definitions, Methods, Psychopathological and Social Outcome', *European Archives of Psychiatry and Neurological Sciences* (in press).

Marneros, A., Steinmeyer, E.M., Deister, A., Rohde, A. and Jünemann, H. (1989b). 'Long-term Outcome of Schizoaffective and Schizophrenic Disorders: A Comparative Study: The Social Consequences', *European Archives of Psychiatry and Neurological Sciences* (in press).

Pickar, D., Roy, A., Breier, A., Doran, A., Wolkowitz, O. Colison, J. and Agren, H. (1986). 'Suicide and Aggression in Schizophrenia: Neurobiological Correlates', *Annals of the New York Academy of Sciences*, 487, 189–96.

Roy, A. (1985). 'Suicide in Psychiatric Patients', *Psychatrica Clinica (North America)*, 8, 227–41.

Steinmeyer, E.M., Marneros, A., Deister, A., Rohde, A. and Jünemann, H. (1989). 'Long-term Outcome of Schizoaffective and Schizophrenic Disorders: A Comparative Study: Causal-analytical Investigations', *European Archives of Psychiatry and Neurological Sciences* (in press).

Schizoaffective disorders and suicidal behaviour: a long-term follow-up study

A. ROHDE, A. MARNERSO and A. DEISTER

Introduction

There have been several studies of suicidal behaviour in schizophrenic or affective disorders, but few investigations in relation to schizoaffective patients. In general the suicide risk in patients with schizoaffective psychoses is considered to be approximately similar to that amongst patients with affective disorders (Angst and Stassen, 1987).

As part of the Cologne Study we investigated the course of the illness and outcome in seventy-two patients with schizoaffective disorders (Marneros *et al.* 1988a–d, 1989a,b; Steinmeyer *et al.* 1989). As one aspect of prognosis, we evaluated suicidal symptomatology and suicidal behaviour during the long-term course of the illness.

Material and methods

The seventy-two patients with schizoaffective psychoses had a mean duration of illness of 25.6 years. The primary population of schizoaffective patients consisted of 108 in-patients in the Cologne University Psychiatric Hospital between 1950 and 1979, diagnosed as 'cases-in-between' (Zwischen-Fälle) according to Kurt Schneider's criteria (1973). The diagnosis 'case-in-between' required a mixture of schizophrenic and affective symptoms. All the cases fulfilled the criteria of schizoaffective disorders used in the Cologne Study (Marneros *et al.* 1986, 1988a), i.e. concurrent or sequential presence of schizophrenic and melancholic or manic symptomatology (DSM-III/DSM-III-R 'Melancholic Type of Major

TABLE 1: Features of study population

Cologne study—schizoaffective disorders (N = 72)			
Sex	female (N = 46)	64%	ratio 1.8:1
	male (N = 26)	36%	
Age at onset (years)			Median = 30.50
			Mean = 32.11
			s.d. = 10.38
			Min. = 15.00
			Max. = 58.00
Age at end of follow-up period (years)			Median = 57.50
			Mean = 57.72
			s.d. = 13.58
			Min. = 27.00
			Max. = 87.00
Duration of follow-up period (years)			Median = 25.00
			Mean = 25.61
			s.d. = 10.46
			Min. = 10.00
			Max. = 59.00
Patients personally interviewed			100%
Place of interview			
— Patients visited us			39%
— Patients were visited at home			57%
— Psychiatric hospital/care unit			4%
Patients' relatives or relevant familiar persons interviewed additionally			57%

Depressive Disorder' and 'Manic Episode', with only slight modifications; for a complete definition see Marneros *et al.* 1988a).

Of the initial group of patients diagnosed as 'cases-in-between' forty-four patients had died; of the sixty-four patients still living, fifty-three were interviewed using the instruments already mentioned in the previous chapter by Rohde *et al.* In addition, nineteen patients of another group diagnosed as cases of 'suspected schizophrenia' on first admission in the same Schneider-oriented clinic were classified as suffering from schizoaffective disorders at follow-up (for criteria considering the longitudinal aspect see Marneros *et al.* 1988a).

Of the forty-four 'cases-in-between' who had died, seven, as far as we know, had committed suicide, i.e. 6.5 per cent of the original group and 16 per cent of the deceased patients. Further investigations on this subject are still being carried out. Table 1 gives information on the seventy-two schizoaffective patients investigated longitudinally.

We evaluated suicidal symptomatology in each patient as well as for every single episode during the whole course of the illness. For statistical evaluation purposes we defined as 'episode' the time between the beginning and the end of in-patient or in-patient-like treatment. In-patient-like treatment was defined in this study as treatment involving: (*a*) intensive medical care (treatment with psychotropic drugs and frequent consultation with a psychiatrist); and (*b*) interruption of usual work or duties.

We recorded attempted suicide separately from suicidal intentions (only thinking about dying or planning to die). However, the results regarding suicidal symptomatology are mainly combined here, because there were no significant differences between suicidal thoughts only and attempted suicide.

Results

Suicidal behaviour in each patient

Nearly two-thirds (65 per cent) of the seventy-two schizoaffective patients had displayed suicidal symptomatology at least once during the course of the illness. More than half of these had become suicidal at least twice. Further analysis shows that 36 per cent of the patients had attempted suicide at least once during the course of the illness, 29 per cent had only had suicidal intentions, and 35 per cent of the patients had never been suicidal.

Comparing suicidal patients and those who had never been suicidal, we found no differences regarding the duration of the illness, the age or marital status at onset or at follow-up, education and vocational training, the social class before and during the illness, and the mean number of episodes.

The only significant difference between suicidal patients and patients who had never been suicidal concerned the sex distribution: 80 per cent of the female patients but only 39 per cent of the male patients had been suicidal at least once.

There was also a highly significant difference between women and men when suicidal intentions and attempted suicide were evaluated separately: 46 per cent of the female, but only 19 per cent of the male patients attempted suicide at least once during the course of the illness, i.e. nearly every second female attempted suicide, but only every fifth male (see Figs. 1 and 2).

Suicidal behaviour in 397 single episodes

Seventy-one schizoaffective patients had 397 episodes (in-patient

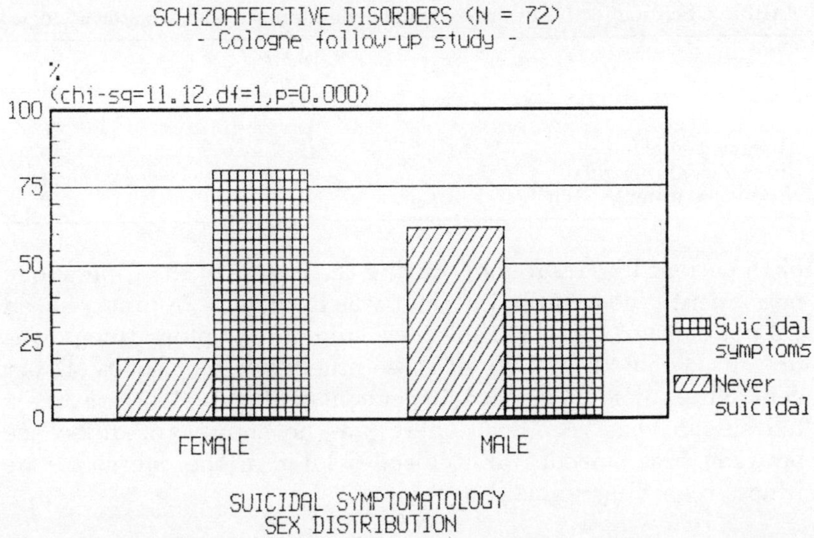

Figure 1: Suicidal symptomatology.

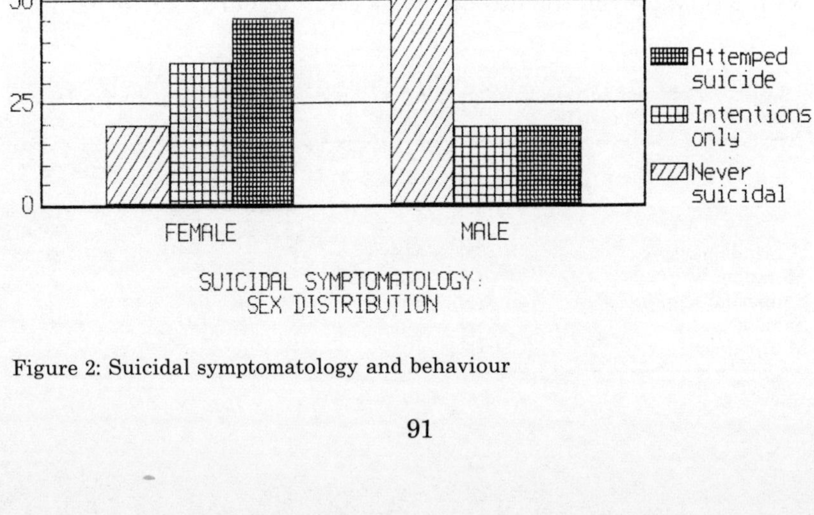

Figure 2: Suicidal symptomatology and behaviour

TABLE 2: Schizoaffective disorders (single episodes): suicidal symptomatology

	Suicidal (N = 97)	*Total (N = 397)*
	%	%
Attempted suicide	41	10
Only suicidal thoughts	59	14
No suicidal symptomatology	–	76

or in-patient-like treatment) during the course of the illness (one permanently hospitalised patient was excluded). In ninety-seven (24 per cent) of these 397 episodes, suicidal symptomatology was present (Table 2). In forty of these ninety-seven episodes (41 per cent of the suicidal episodes, 10 per cent of all episodes) an attempted suicide was recorded. There was no significant difference between first episodes and episodes later in the course of the illness regarding suicidal behaviour.

Intrasymptomatological factors in episodes

In 61 per cent of our schizoaffective patients the course of the illness was polymorphous, i.e. they suffered from different types of episodes during the course of the illness (schizodepressive, schizomanic, schizomanic-depressive, melancholic, manic, manic-depressive, schizophrenic, non-characteristic; definitions in Marneros *et al.* 1986a, 1988a, 1988d). In only 39 per cent of the patients was the course of the illness monomorphous, i.e. the episode was always of the same type, mostly schizodepressive. The highest rate of suicidal symptomatology (42 per cent) was found in schizodepressive episodes, i.e. episodes with a concurrent presence of schizophrenic and melancholic symptoms. In patients who had had schizodepressive episodes, the percentage of patients with suicidal symptomatology was even higher than in patients

TABLE 3: Schizoaffective disorders (single episodes): suicidal symptomatology in different types of episode

		Suicidal symptoms	*Attempted suicide*
		%	%
Schizodepressive	(N = 165)	42	19
Melancholic	(N = 36)	25	8
Schizomanic-depressive	(N = 53)	21	8
Schizophrenic	(N = 29)	17	3
Manic-depressive	(N = 10)	10	–

TABLE 4: Schizoaffective disorders (single episodes): groups of episodes and suicidal symptomatology

		Suicidal symptoms	*Attempted suicide*
		%	%
Schizoaffective episodes	(N = 294)	28	12
Affective episodes	(N = 58)	17	5
Schizophrenic	(N = 29)	17	3

who had suffered from melancholic episodes (25 per cent; Table 3). The percentage of patients with suicidal symptoms in schizophrenic episodes is very nearly the same as that in the hospitalised cases in the schizophrenic population (see also previous chapter). The highest percentage of attempted suicide (19 per cent, Table 3) also occurs in schizodepressive episodes.

For schizoaffective (schizodepressive, schizomanic, schizomanic-depressive) episodes a higher rate of suicidal symptomatology was found than in pure affective (melancholic, manic, manic-depressive) or pure schizophrenic episodes (Table 4). In 34 per cent of all episodes with a depressive component (schizodepressive, melancholic, manic-depressive, schizomanic-depressive) suicidal behaviour was recorded.

The presence or absence of productive psychotic symptomatology in general was not found to influence the frequency of suicidal symptomatology. The presence or absence of delusions or hallucinations in general or of paranoid-hallucinatory syndromes was also not significant. But there were some important differences regarding some single symptoms (Table 5): episodes with suicidal behaviour have significantly more acoustic hallucinations than episodes without suicidality, more mood-congruent delusions, and more first-rank symptoms. This means that symptoms not

TABLE 5: Schizoaffective disorders (single episodes): psychopathology

	No suicidal symptoms (N = 300)	*Suicidal (N = 97)*	*Total (N = 397)*
	%	%	%
Acoustic hallucinations	8*	*16*	10
Mood-congruent delusions	3**	*14*	6
First-rank symptoms	7**	*18*	10
Incoherence	17	*14*	16

chi-square-test: ** = $p < 0.01$, * = $p < 0.05$.

necessarily connected with depressive mood, i.e. first-rank symptoms, also seem to promote suicidal behaviour.

Extrasymptomatological factors at time of episode

We also investigated whether several extrasymptomatological factors differentiate suicidal and non-suicidal episodes. No differences regarding the season of admission or the presence of stressful life events were found between the suicidal and non-suicidal groups.

We found differences regarding marital status at the time of the episode, but not those we had expected (Table 6). Married patients were over-represented in the group of suicidal episodes (76 per cent, 60 per cent of total episodes) whilst single patients had less suicidal episodes (11 per cent) than the total group (23 per cent).

Another interesting factor is the employment situation at the time of the episode. Table 7 shows that housewives are over-represented in the group of suicidal episodes (51 per cent). Being unemployed or retired was not very frequent in suicidal episodes;

TABLE 6: Schizoaffective disorders (single episodes): marital state at time of episode

Marital state	*No suicidal symptoms (N = 300)*	*Suicidal (N = 97)*	*Total (N = 397)*
	%	%	%
Single	27	11	23
Married	54	76	60
Separated/Divorced	15	8	13
Widowed	4	4	4

$X^2 = 15.75$, df = 3, $p < 0.01$

TABLE 7: Schizoaffective disorders (single episodes): occupational state at time of episode

Occupational state	*No suicidal symptoms (N = 300)*	*Suicidal (N = 97)*	*Total (N = 397)*
	%	%	%
Employed	58	37	53
Unemployed	2	1	2
Housewife	26	51	32
Retired	3	3	3
Retired early (because of psychiatric illness)	11	8	10

$X^2 = 20.07$, df = 4, $p < 0.001$

TABLE 8: Schizoaffective disorders (single episodes): method of attempted suicide

Method of attempted suicide	*Attempted suicide (N = 40)*
	%
Drug intoxication	62.5
Jumping out of the window	12.5
Poisoning	5.0
Gas	2.5
Cutting artery	2.5
Cutting throat	2.5
Combination of several methods/other methods	12.5

being employed, at 37 per cent, is less frequent in the total group of episodes.

Methods of attempted suicide

Table 8 shows the methods used in attempted suicide. In nearly two-thirds (62.5 per cent) of the cases drugs or pills were taken. The next most common method (12.5 per cent) was jumping out of the window. Other methods used were poisoning (5 per cent), cutting (5 per cent) and gas (2.5 per cent). So-called 'soft' methods were more frequent (67.5 per cent) than 'hard' methods (22.5 per cent).

Suicidality in intervals

Suicidal symptoms outside periods of acute exacerbation of the illness were seldom found, in contrast to our schizophrenic population (see previous chapter by Rohde *et al.*).

Conclusions

The present investigation confirms the findings of other authors that schizoaffective patients are at high risk for suicidal symptomatology (Angst, 1980, 1987; Dingman and McGlashan, 1986; Cohen *et al.* 1972; Omata, 1985). In the Cologne Study, 65 per cent of the schizoaffective patients displayed suicidal symptoms at least once during the course of the illness. Amongst schizoaffective patients, females are much more likely than males (80 per cent compared with 39 per cent) both to have suicidal thoughts and to attempt suicide (49 per cent compared with 19 per cent).

Evaluating single episodes of in-patient or in-patient-like treatment, we found that 24 per cent of them were suicidal. The highest frequency of suicidality was found in patients with schizodepressive episodes (42 per cent), followed by those with melancholic (25 per cent), schizomanic-depressive (21 per cent), and schizophrenic episodes (17 per cent). Significantly more acoustic hallucinations, mood-congruent delusions and first-rank symptoms were recorded amongst patients with suicidal episodes.

Marital status and occupational status at the time of the episode seem to be important to a certain degree: being married and being a housewife seems to increase the risk of suicidal behaviour. Further investigations on the importance of such factors as sex, marital status, occupational status, and type of episode are currently being carried out.

There was no difference between suicidal and non-suicidal episodes regarding age of the patient at the time of the episode, the presence or absence of residual symptoms, and whether it was the first episode or a later episode in the course of the illness. In nearly every second episode an attempted suicide was recorded, mostly with so-called 'soft' methods such as intoxication with pills.

References

American Psychiatric Association (1980). *Diagnostic and Statistical Manual of Mental Disorders*, 3rd edn, Washington: APA.

—— (1987). *Diagnostic and Statistical Manual of Mental Disorders*, 3rd edn (revised), Washington: APA.

Angst, J. (1980) 'Verlauf unipolar depressiver, bipolar manischdepressiver und schizo-affektiver Erkrankungen und Psychosen', *Fortschritte Neurologie Psychiatrie*, 48, 3–30.

—— (1987). 'Epidemiologie der affektiven Psychosen', in K.P. Kisker, H. Lauter, J.E. Meyer, C. Müller and C. Strömgren (eds.), *Psychiatrie der Gegenwart*, 3rd edn, vol. 5, Springer.

—— and Stassen, H.H. (1987). 'Verlaufsaspekte affektiver Psychosen: Suizide, Rückfallrisiko im Alter', in G. Huber (ed.), *Fortschritte in der Psychosenforschung*, Schattauer.

Cohen, S.M., Allen, M.G., Pollin, W. and Hrubec, Z. (1972). 'Relationship of Schizo-Affective Psychosis to Manic Depressive Psychosis and Schizophrenia', *Archives of General Psychiatry*, 26, 539–46.

Dingman, C. and McGlashan, T. (1986). 'Discriminating Characteristics of Suicides', *Acta Psychiatrica Scandinavica*, 74, 91–7.

Marneros, A., Deister, A. and Rohde, A. (1986). 'The Cologne Study on Schizoaffective Disorders and Schizophrenia Suspects', in A. Marneros and M.T. Tsuang (eds.), *Schizoaffective Psychoses*, Springer.

—— Jünemann, H. and Fimmers, R. (1988a). 'Long-term Course of Schizoaffective Disorders: Definitions, Methods, Frequency of Episodes and Cycles', *European Archives of Psychiatry and Neurological Sciences*, 237, 264–75.

—— (1988b). 'Long-term Course of Schizoaffective Disorders: Length of Cycles, Episodes and Intervals', *European Archives of Psychiatry and Neurological Sciences*, 237, 276–82.

—— (1988c). 'Long-term Course of Schizoaffective Disorders: Onset, Type of Episodes and Syndrome Shift, Precipitating Factors, Suicidality, Inactivity of Illness and Outcome', *European Archives of Psychiatry and Neurological Sciences*, 237, 283–90.

Marneros, A., Rohde, A., Deister, A. and Jünemann, H. (1988d) 'Syndrome Shift in Long-term Course of Schizoaffective Disorders', *European Archives of Psychiatry and Neurological Sciences* (in press).

Marneros, A., Deister, A., Rohde, A., Steinmeyer, E.M. and Jünemann, H. (1989a). 'Long-term Outcome of Schizoaffective and Schizophrenic Disorders: A Comparative Study: Definitions, Methods, Psychopathological and Social Outcome', *European Archives of Psychiatry and Neurological Sciences* (in press).

Marneros, A., Steinmeyer, E.M., Deister, A., Rohde, A. and Jünemann, H. (1989b). 'Long-term Outcome of Schizoaffective and Schizophrenic Disorders: A Comparative Study: The Social Consequences', *European Archives of Psychiatry and Neurological Sciences* (in press).

Omata, W. (1985). 'Schizoaffektive Psychosen in Deutschland und in Japan—eine transkulturell-psychiatrische Studie', *Fortschritte Neurologie Psychiatrie*, 53, 168–76.

Rohde, A., Marneros, A. and Deister, A. (1989a). 'Suicidal Behaviour in Schizophrenic Patients—a Follow-up Investigation', in N. Kreitman and S. Platt (eds.), *Proceedings of the Second European Symposium on Suicidal Behaviour*, Edinburgh University Press.

Rohde, A. and Marneros, A. (1989b). 'Suizidalität bei schizoaffektiven Psychosen', in A. Marneros (ed.), *Diagnose, Therapie und Prophylaxe der schizoaffektiven Psychosen*, Springer.

Schneider, K. (1973). *Clinical Psychopathology*, New York: Grune and Stratton.

Steinmeyer, E.M., Marneros, A., Deister, A., Rohde, A. and Jünemann, H. (1989). 'Long-term Outcome of Schizoaffective and Schizophrenic Disorders: A Comparative Study: Casual-analytical Investigations', *European Archives of Psychiatry and Neurological Sciences* (in press).

4

SOCIAL AND PSYCHOPATHOLOGICAL ASPECTS OF PARASUICIDE

Deliberate self-poisoning: a symptom of deprivation

M. DALY, M.J. KELLEHER, B. KEOHANE, C. LINEHAN and W. LORENZ

There have been numerous investigations into the different aspects of non-fatal deliberate self-poisoning, a problem which has increased rapidly and progressively over the last three and a half decades, and which currently absorbs a very large proportion of medical and psychiatric time and resources.

One type of investigation has been the ecological study, the purpose of which is to isolate the factors which contribute to the increase of deliberate self-poisoning by identifying the characteristics of the neighbourhoods in which it flourishes.

Ecological studies have been carried out in a number of cities in Britain: in Bristol (Morgan *et al.* 1975); in Oxford (Bancroft *et al.*. 1975); and Edinburgh (Holding *et al.* 1977). These studies ranked the electoral wards of these cities according to their rates of suicide attempts and then correlated them with indices of social disorganisation. The studies consistently showed a strong association between high rates of deliberate self-harm and disorganised central city areas with overcrowding, lack of basic amenities, and an over-representation of social classes four and five. A very high percentage of social problems also characterised these wards, with marital disharmony, alcoholism, trouble with the law, juvenile delinquency, and cruelty to children.

In 1982, a similar study carried out in Cork (Daly *et al.* 1986) identified three distinct types of neighbourhood in which these non-fatal acts occurred most frequently. First, there were the local authority housing estates built some thirty years ago with the intention of rehousing slum dwellers. The children in these wards have grown to be adults, sometimes into single parents, sometimes married and living with their spouse and children in their parents' home. In consequence, there is serious overcrowding in these wards. Secondly, we had very extensive housing estates built on the periphery of the city. These had been developed over the previous decade and a half to provide inexpensive accommodation for families at an early stage of development. These families often felt very isolated. The development of community facilities was slow and the lack of adequate public transport meant that visits to relatives and former friends was difficult for parents of young children.

Thirdly, self-poisoning occurred frequently in parts of the city centre where large, old houses had been divided up to provide rented accommodation for single people, and in areas where the hostels for the homeless were situated.

Altogether 243 people from Cork City were treated in hospital following a deliberate act of self-poisoning in 1982. Twenty-seven (just over 10 per cent) repeated the overdose at least once in 1982. The proportion of Irish males involved in self-poisoning was 44 per cent—much higher than in the British studies. Only 27 per cent of the self-poisoners in Cork in 1982 were young people taking an overdose as a result of an interpersonal problem. For the rest, social problems, problems due to alcoholism and the difficulties of living in very deprived material circumstances were important predisposing factors.

The aims of the present study were to build up a detailed picture of the social matrix of the city from details of the 1981 census and to estimate the extent of social distress from the records of the community care workers so that electoral wards ranked high and low for self-poisoning in the 1982 study could be compared according to a number of epidemiological factors. Secondly, we wished to see whether the age structure and stage of family development of a ward had a bearing on the rate of self-poisoning; in other words, to see whether a very large proportion of young women and girls in a ward might result in a high rate of self-poisoning, irrespective of social conditions. The final aim was to follow up and interview all of those identified in the original study, beginning with the twenty-seven individuals who repeated the act of self-poisoning at least once in 1982. The first stage of the follow-up study has been completed.

Method

A computer program was designed for the electoral wards of the city. Details of the population structure were obtained from the

1981 census on eight variables. These were the population density and the size of the households, the age, sex and stage of family development in the ward, the marital and employment status, and the level of education reached by the inhabitants of each ward. The rates of Deliberate Overdose (DOD) for the city were taken from a previous study by the authors. The Community Care records were studied and details obtained of the number of referrals and the type of social problems in each ward.

Because differences in self-poisoning rates between wards could be the result of population factors such as the age of the inhabitants or the characteristics of the ward (such as whether it was used predominantly for business or domiciliary purposes), we examined the status of each ward with regard to the eight variables on the computer program and compared the wards with high rates of self-poisoning with wards built in the same period of time and with a very similar structure but with much lower rates of DOD.

The first stage of the follow up study was to trace and interview the twenty-seven individuals who repeated the overdose in 1982: twenty-six were traced; twenty were interviewed directly; relatives and social workers gave details of the remainder.

Results

In 1982, 243 people were treated in hospital following a deliberate overdose (DOD). This gave an average city rate of 178 per 100 000 population. However, the rates for the different electoral wards of the city varied widely (Figure 1). Churchfield, the highest ranking ward had a rate of 745 per 100 000; Knocknaheeney, the second highest had a rate of 543 per 100 000; while the lowest ranking wards had rates of 60, 63, and 67 per 100 000, respectively. There were high rates of DOD both in the local authority housing estates on the periphery of the city and in parts of the city centre.

Table 1 shows the type and percentage of referrals to the community care services of those wards with high rates of DOD. Marital problems, including conflict, separation, desertion, and unmarried mothers in distress make up the greatest proportion of these. These problems were the primary reason for contacting Community Care, but in many cases several factors contributed to each referral. The percentage of calls concerned with alcoholism is rather low. However, it is often not the alcoholic but another family member (usually the spouse) who contacts the services,

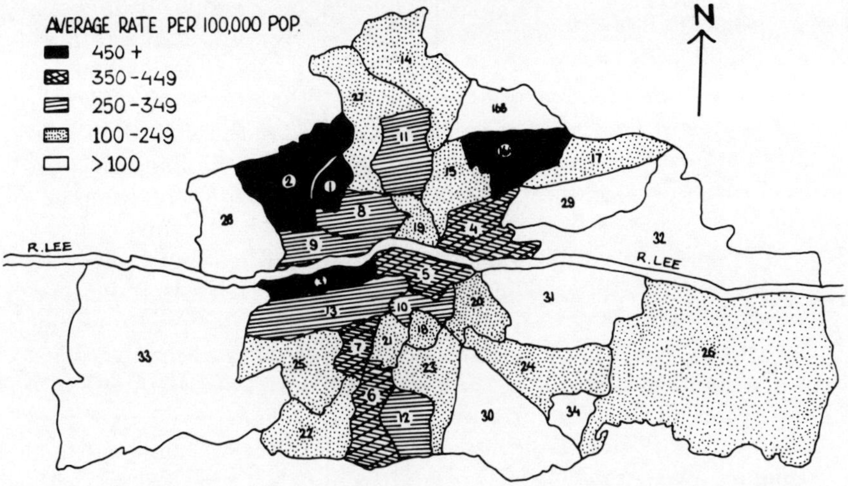

Figure 1: Deliberate overdose rates (DOD) in Cork City Wards, 1982

and the problems are then classified under marital problems rather than alcohol problems.

Table 2 shows the correlation of DOD with referrals to Community Care. Marital problems, housing difficulties, alcoholism, and child neglect all correlate strongly with self-poisoning, but, interestingly enough, financial difficulties correlate only very weakly with the problem. This suggests that overcrowding and interpersonal difficulties are much more stressful than poverty alone.

Table 3 shows the wards we compared, the high-rated local authority housing estates and similar wards, composed mainly of housing estates built in the same period of time for young families

TABLE 1: Social referrals: Cork City wards with high rates of DOD

	Churchfield	*Knocknaheeney*	*The Glen*	*Mayfield*
Marital problems	11	37	27	30
Housing problems	6	4	4	3
Alcoholism	5	7	5	13
Child neglect	4	10	7	11
Financial difficulties	1	3	11	9
Rate for ward	12.7	10.1	18.3	13.2

TABLE 2: Correlation (r) of DOD with social distress variables

Marital problems	*Alcoholism*	*Child neglect*	*Debts*	*Housing difficulties*
r = 0.47 p = 0.01	r = 0.33 p = 0.03	r = 0.35 p = 0.02	r = 0.02 p = NS	r = 0.38 p = 0.01

TABLE 3: Names and periods of development of the wards compared

High rates	*Low rates*	*Data developed*
Churchfield	Ballinlough B & C	1966–75
Mayfield	Bishopstown C & E	1965–75
Knocknaheeney	Tivoli B	1970–80
The Glen B		

in an early stage of development, but with low rates of self-poisoning. The high-rated wards had a slight excess of males.

Table 4 shows the differences found between the wards rated high and low for self-poisoning. The high-rated wards were almost entirely composed of local authority housing estates. The low-rated wards were mostly owner occupied. The high-rated wards had larger families. Over 35 per cent of the population was under fourteen years in the high-rated wards, compared with 25 per cent or less in the low-rated wards. In Knocknaheeney the families were particularly large; 50 per cent of the population was under fourteen years. There was greater overcrowding in the high-rated wards; an average of 0.92 persons per room as against 0.63; and there was a greater density of people in the high-rated wards: 50–85 persons per hectare compared with 26–35 in the low-rated wards. Unemployment was much higher in the high-rated wards: 13–24 per cent compared with 2.5–8 per cent in the low-rated wards; and there was a great discrepancy between the amount of education received in both types of wards. Between 24 per cent and 48 per cent of the 15–29-year-olds stopped their education at fourteen years in the high-rated wards, only 3–6 per cent did so in

TABLE 4: Comparison between wards

	High-rated wards	*Low-rated wards*
Housing tenure	70–90% (LA housing)	< 70% (owner occupied)
Family size	> 35% (pop. age 0–14)	< 26% (pop. age 0–14)
Overcrowding	0.92 (persons per room)	0.63 (persons per room)
Persons per hectare	50–85	26–36
Unemployment	13.5–24%	2.5–8%
Education (stopped at fourteen years)	24–48% (15–29-year-olds)	3–6% (15–29-year-olds)
Social referrals	10–16.3 (per 1000 pop.)	1.9–3.2 (per 1000 pop.)

TABLE 5: Differences between self-poisoners in the city centre and local authority housing estates

	City centre	*Housing estates*
	%	%
Sex	60 male	36 male
Marital status	74 single	33 single
Living alone	60	2
Repeated changes of address	30	10
Personality disorder	44	15
Severe social problems	52	28

the low-rated wards. Finally, referrals for social problems were 10–16.5 per 1000 population in the high-rated wards compared with 1.9–3.2 per 1000 population in the low-rated wards.

Table 5 shows some of the characteristics of self-poisoners in the city centre and contrasts these with the local authority housing estates. The self-poisoners in the city centre were more likely to be single men, living alone with no fixed abode: 52 per cent had severe social problems and 44 per cent had severe personality disorders.

Table 6 gives some of the characteristics of those who repeated the DOD in 1982. Twenty-six of the twenty-seven were traced. These were thirteen males and thirteen females. The one untraced was a male drug addict. Only five were married, the rest were

TABLE 6: Characteristics of those who repeated the DOD (N = 27)

Characteristic	*Number*
Sex	
male	14
female	13
Marital status	
married	5
single	15
married but separated	6
widowed	1
Psychiatric disturbance	
alcohol problems	16
drug addicts	2
gross personality disorders	7
low IQ	6
Family history of severe psychiatric disturbance	6
Chronic material deprivation	12
Accumulation of life events	5

Table 7: Duration of suicidal behaviour

- In 2 cases death followed a subsequent overdose less than a year after the study.
- In 3 cases the suicidal behaviour occurred over a brief period and was never subsequently repeated.
- In 7 cases the suicidal behaviour continued for 2–4 years but was discontinued because of improved personal circumstances.
- In 15 cases the suicidal behaviour is ongoing.

single or married but separated; one was widowed. There was a high level of psychiatric morbidity and six had a family history of severe psychiatric disturbance, with suicide and suicidal behaviour among the first-degree family members. Twelve lived in very poor material circumstances, only in five cases were external events alone thought to have precipitated the suicidal behaviour.

Table 7 shows the duration of suicidal behaviour in those who repeated the DOD in 1982. In most cases the suicidal behaviour continues or has resulted in death following an overdose less than a year after the study. In only ten cases has the suicidal behaviour been discontinued.

Discussion

This study confirms what others have demonstrated, that self-poisoning most frequently occurs in areas of social deprivation and disorganisation. The only surprising finding was the strength of the correlation found in Cork City.

The contrast in social conditions between the high-rated and low-rated wards was very marked. Those wards with the highest rates of self-poisoning had also the most severe overcrowding in the city and the greatest number of social problems, more marital conflict, separation and desertion, more child neglect and cruelty to children, more alcoholism and trouble with the law. The level of education reached in the two wards with the highest rates of self-poisoning was extremely low compared with the rest of the city. Over 40 per cent of the 15–29 year olds had finished their education at fourteen years, compared with less than 30 per cent in all wards of the city, and only 3–6 per cent in the low-rated wards. A point of interest here is the fact that less than 10 per cent of the population of the housing estates with high rates on the periphery of the city is over forty-five years old, in fact less than 30 per cent is over thirty. This means that the lack of formal education is compounded by the fact that there are few older relatives and friends to give support and advice to the young parents.

Unemployment correlated strongly with self-poisoning in both studies: 44 per cent of those interviewed in the first study were unemployed, though only four gave it as the reason for taking the overdose. In the second study the unemployment rate was 13–24 per cent in the wards rated high for DOD, compared with 2.5–8 per cent in the low-rated wards. All of the follow-up group whose suicidal behaviour continues were unemployed.

Platt (1984) has suggested that unemployment may be important as a predisposing and vulnerability factor, increasing family tensions, isolating individuals, and leading to depression, hopelessness, and the misuse of alcohol.

The self-poisoners in the city centre were mostly single people who lived in flats or bedsitters or in the hostels for the homeless. Many had been excluded from their family home on account of their behaviour and, with no permanent address, they lived at times in hostels for the homeless, at times in mental hospitals or prisons, and at other times stayed with acquaintances for a few weeks. The majority were well known to the psychiatric services and a considerable number had severe personality disorders. They appeared to have greater difficulties in terms of social and forensic problems and in their basic personality than the residents of the housing estates, who were more likely to be living with their families and suffering the social stresses of overcrowding, marital conflict, and bringing up children without adequate support.

Most of the repeaters were a very vulnerable group. In only three cases did the suicidal behaviour continue over a brief period of time, in response to adverse circumstances, never subsequently to be repeated. In a further seven cases, the suicidal behaviour continued over a period of two to four years and has not been repeated since. These people describe the significant impact of outside intervention in their lives, such as the successful treatment of alcoholism and stable community living and activity.

For the majority of patients, the suicidal behaviour continues. Most live in very poor material circumstances and their personal resources are inadequate to permit them to escape. The suicidal behaviour appears to be associated with sudden or periodic deterioration of material circumstances and life events which are overwhelmingly stressful to this group and which frequently precipitate a suicide attempt. All of these received in-patient treatment at the time of the overdose, but they described ambivalent relationships with the professional services, complaining that their whole situation had never been fully taken into account.

Conclusion

Cork City has a serious self-poisoning problem associated with a deprived environment, local authority housing, unemployment, interpersonal stress, and child neglect. The level of educational achievements in the high-rated wards is low and young people may feel a sense of powerlessness when trying to control their lives or change difficult circumstances.

What should be done to reduce the distress and self-poisoning which is a sign of the distress in these deprived areas? Should it be better material conditions and a different mix of population? Better infrastructure and a more broadly based education system? Should it be more social workers and community leaders? It is obvious that the ordinary medical model is inadequate to meet the needs of people living in these deprived conditions.

References

Bancroft, J.H.J., Skrimshire, A., Reynold, F., Simkins, and Smith, J. (1975). 'Self-poisoning and Self-injury in the Oxford area: Epidemiological Aspects, 1969–73', *British Journal of Preventive & Social Medicine*, 29, 170–7.

Daly, M., Conway, M. and Kelleher, M.J. (1986). 'Social Determinants of Self-Poisoning', *British Journal of Psychiatry*, 148, 406–13.

Holding, T.A., Buglass, D., Duffy, J.C. and Kreitman, N. (1977). Parasuicide in Edinburgh—A Seven-Year Review 1968–1974, *British Journal of Psychiatry* 130, 534–43.

Morgan, H.G., Pocock, H. and Pottle, S. (1975). 'The urban distribution of non-fatal deliberate self-harm', *British Journal of Psychiatry*, 126, 319–328.

Platt, S. (1984). 'Unemployment and Suicidal Behaviour: A Review of the Literature', *Social Science & Medicine*, 19 (2), 93–115.

Field dependence and dichotomous thinking in patients who have attempted suicide: traits or state variables?

ARMIN SCHMIDTKE, SYLVIA SCHALLER, EVELYN FLURSCHÜTZ and GERD MEIER

Problem

In attempting to explain suicidal behaviour, hypotheses suggesting that certain cognitive styles may be peculiar to suicidal persons have often been put forward, the assumption being that their attitudes and behaviour are 'illogical'. It has been claimed that such persons exhibit deficient cognitive capabilities, and that their thinking is characterised by narrowness, rigidity, and inflexibility, as well as by an 'either/or' approach to situations, e.g. an inability to distinguish the essential from the inessential, or inappropriate retrieval strategies for autobiographical memories (Neuringer, 1964; Rothe, 1980; Schrader *et al.*, 1986; Williams and Broadbent, 1986). If this is indeed the case, such an outlook may well result in the false evaluation of situations or events which may be of a potentially suicide-triggering nature. Also, erroneous suicide-provoking attitudes towards life and death have often been explained in terms of inadequate cognition (Orbach and Glaubman, 1978).

In spite of such assertions, most previous investigations of the intelligence and/or intelligence structure of suicidal persons have revealed that both adolescent and adult suicides and parasuicides, in general, exhibit intelligence values not significantly different from those observable in control groups. Even when comparisons were made within the same diagnostic groups, only very few investigations revealed lower values for patients who had attempted suicide.

The discrepancies between the results of previous studies can be explained, at least partly, by inadequate methodologies, unsatisfactory approaches, and deficient sample-matching.

However, closer inspection of such results reveals that, although suicidal persons are usually virtually indistinguishable from control groups with respect to estimates of their global intelligence or their verbal performance, they do perform less well in non-verbal tasks (processes) and in situations which test problem-solving abilities (Smith, 1981). The findings obtained by such testing, which gives a more accurate insight into cognitive styles, would appear to support the hypothesis that suicidal behaviour (at least in the case of parasuicides) results from inadequacy with respect to problem-solving. Furthermore, in tests designed to assess fluid intelligence (according to Cattell's definition) as opposed to verbal intelligence (so-called crystallised intelligence), lower values have been reported for suicidal patients (e.g. Levenson and Neuringer, 1971; Eastwood *et al.*, 1972).

On the basis of the findings discussed so far, there would seem to be little point in prolonging efforts to demonstrate that global intelligence and general cognitive capability are factors which may condition suicidal acts. Instead, a worthwhile approach would appear to be that of identifying particular cognitive styles which are specific, or predisposing, to suicidal behaviour. In the present study, we focused on two such cognitive styles: namely, field dependence and dichotomous thinking.

Neuringer was one of the first investigators to attempt an empirical demonstration of dichotomous thinking in suicidal patients. In support of this hypothesis some studies (Neuringer, 1961, 1967; Neuringer and Lettieri, 1982) have demonstrated significant differences among suicidal persons, psychiatric patients, and controls; in some cases, for all three factors of the semantic differential significant results were found. However, in some studies, the dichotomous thinking of suicides was found to be not significantly different from that of psychiatric patients. Wetzel (1975), using semantic-differential assessments of dichotomous thinking, was also unable to detect significant differences between patients with different suicidal tendencies.

With respect to field dependence, it appears that Witkin's hypotheses may also be of particular relevance to suicide research. According to his theory (Witkin *et al.*, 1971, 1979), certain types of behaviour covary with, or are functionally related to, a person's ability to differentiate. Thus, field-independent persons are supposed to be more capable than field-dependent individuals of distinguishing nuances in the forms of expression or opinions of other people. Those exhibiting field dependence are more easily affected by, and are more aware of, social stimuli. On the other hand, they may have poor discriminative abilities with regard to the importance of certain social stimuli and may, therefore, be less socially perceptive and more dependent on their social environment. As a result, field-dependent persons may be more oriented towards interpersonal contacts and enjoy social situations more than field-independent persons (Witkin and Goodenough, 1977).

Also, with respect to the use of defence and coping mechanisms in the event of conflict and stress, it is supposed that field-dependent and field-independent persons exhibit differences, with the former being more affected by stressful events.

In extreme manifestations of this cognitive style, differences with respect to types of psychic illnesses have been reported, with persons whose values are at the two extremes of this dimension exhibiting a higher prevalence of psychopathologic syndromes than persons with more moderate values (Parkes, 1981).

On the basis of these findings, Levenson (1974) put forward the hypothesis that, under certain conditions, limited conceptualisation faculties increase the probability of psychopathological deviation and, from a certain point (possibly a threshold), the likelihood of suicidal behaviour. He further emphasised that this possibility is not merely confined to affective behaviour.

The dimension, field dependence versus field independence, has also been discussed previously within the framework of other personality theories (Eysenck, 1967). Fine (1972) compared field-dependent introverts with the 'overcontrolled individual' as defined by Megargee (Megargee, 1967; Megargee *et al.*, 1967) and believed that, in individuals with this combination of traits, a higher frequency of sudden outbreaks of aggression is likely to be encountered.

However, objections can still be raised to such results, and the hypotheses stemming from them, on the grounds that it is impossible to rule out the validity of the opposing hypothesis which suggests that the differences measured in such tests could be attributable to cerebral dysfunction, this being perhaps the result of the suicide attempt itself (e.g. stemming from the intoxication, Eastwood *et al.*, 1972). Moreover, the influence of medication (e.g. from therapeutic counter-measures) also needs to be taken into account. Unfortunately, specific detailed investigations of this aspect are not yet available.

It also remains uncertain whether the findings mentioned

above are specific to suicidal patients. Thus, the validity of the conclusion drawn by Neuringer in 1961, that this cognitive style represents a general correlate of emotional disturbance rather than of suicidal behaviour, remains an open question (see also Neuringer, 1974). For example, it is conceivable that this form of thinking emerges and is applied only in crises (Lester, 1970). This would explain why the threshold barrier, 'fear of death', is switched off (Spiegel and Neuringer, 1963). Therefore, a dichotomy exists between the assumption that these cognitive styles are personality factors and the perspective that maintains that these cognitive styles are task-specific, i.e. behavioural phenomena observable only under certain conditions.

The aim of the present study was, therefore, to investigate whether, apart from general differences between patients after a suicide attempt and other psychiatric patients, these cognitive styles can, in suicidal persons, be considered as traits rather than as state variables.

Study

Design

To investigate this question, the overall strategy employed was a longitudinal design that could best be termed an extended Solomon fourfold design. Each patient was tested three times: first, within three days after the suicide attempt; secondly, when possible, eighteen to twenty-one days after the first testing; and finally, at the time of discharge from hospital. Discharge was taken to indicate 'improvement'.

To control for whether the effects observed were dependent on the repetition of the test and/or the time of testing (i.e. the time period elapsing between admission and first testing), we began the testing at varying points in time in certain randomly chosen cases.

Samples and methods

Table 1 gives information concerning the size and composition of the sample groups. These comprised patients who, after a suicide attempt, had been transferred to a psychiatric institute for in-patient treatment, as well as other psychiatric patients. Most were voluntary admissions. For comparison, we used a random sample of psychiatric controls. For methodological reasons, we matched, in an additional step, the psychiatric controls with

TABLE 1: Sample sizes and diagnoses

	Males			*Females*		
	Parasuicides	*Psychiatric controls (random)*	*Psychiatric controls (matched)*	*Parasuicides*	*Psychiatric controls (random)*	*Psychiatric controls (matched)*
N	28	52	28	28	73	28
Mean age	33.78	37.77	34.26	37.35	37.62	36.58
ICD diagnosis	(Percentages)	Percentages	(Percentages)	(Percentages)	(Percentages)	(Percentages)
296						
Manic-depressive psychosis, manic		4.08	3.70		8.95	
Manic-depressive psychosis. depr.	16.67	34.69	29.63	26.92	34.33	29.63
Other					2.99	3.70
295						
Schizophrenic psychosis	16.67	10.20	18.52	7.69	20.90	25.93
297						
Paranoid states	4.17					
298						
Non-organic psychosis, depr.		2.04	3.70	3.85	1.49	3.70
300						
Neurotic disorders	4.17	8.16	11.11		4.48	7.41
Neurotic depression	25.00	10.20	14.81	30.77	4.48	3.70

301 + 302 Personality disord. Sexual deviations	8.33	14.28	11.11	7.69	8.96	14.81
303–305 Alcohol and drug-related diagnoses	4.17	8.16		3.85	2.99	3.70
306 + 307 Pysiological malfunction Special symptoms		4.08	3.70		7.46	3.70
308 + 309 Acute reaction to stress Adjustment reaction	20.83	4.08	3.70	19.23	1.49	
310 Nonpsychotic disorders follow. CD					1.49	3.70

regard to age and sex. The frequency of the occurrence of certain diagnoses according to ICD-9 changed after the matching. Due to the specific psychiatric diagnoses linked with suicidal behaviour (ICD 308 and 309)—'contaminated diagnoses'—it was not possible to match the groups totally with regard to diagnoses.

To measure intelligence we used an abridged German version of the Wechsler Adult Intelligence Scale, with verbal and performance subtests. To measure fluid intelligence we applied the Standard Progressive Matrices Test (Raven, 1971).

To measure dichotomous thinking we followed Neuringer in using a semantic differential: in our study, this consisted of thirty-seven scales. Patients were asked to judge the concepts, 'self', 'ideal self', 'negative self', 'looking-glass self family', and 'looking-glass self environment', as well as the colour 'white'. Our reason for including this last concept was that it should be as neutral as possible and totally unrelated to the persons questioned.

We evaluated the occurrence of extreme answers—segregated according to their positive or negative direction—in relation to the number of possible answers as well as to the frequency of answers belonging to the neutral middle category.

To measure field dependence, we applied our own German version of the Group Embedded Figures Test (Schmidtke and Schaller, 1987).

Results

Figure 1 shows the results obtained with respect to intelligence scores. We found no significant differences between either the sexes or the different clinical groups in the verbal and performance scores in the Wechsler scales, or in the mean values for the Standard Progressive Matrices.

Figure 2 shows the results obtained with respect to field dependence. The values for the suicidal patients and the psychiatric controls did not differ significantly, but we did find significant differences with regard to sex.

An analysis of variance, including values for normal controls —the factors were clinical classification (suicide attempts, psychiatric controls, normal persons) and sex—revealed significance with regard to the factor clinical classification. However, the *a posteriori* test showed that this significance was due only to the difference between, on the one hand, the suicidal and psychiatric group, and, on the other, the normal controls (Table 2). With

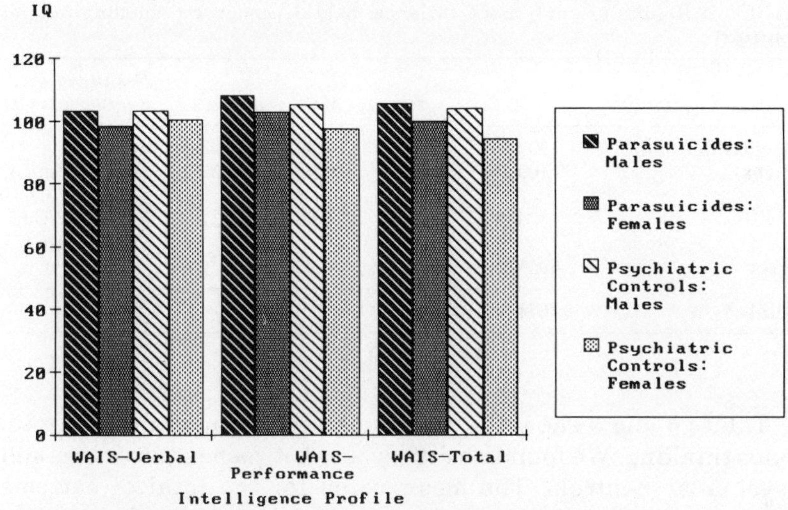

Figure 1: Intelligence profiles of tested groups.

regard to the results of repeated measurements, a split plot analysis of variance yielded significant results also for the factor 'repeated measurement' and a significant effect for the interaction sex × measurement. This effect remained significant even after the degrees of freedom had been corrected according to the procedure of Greenhouse and Geisser (Table 3).

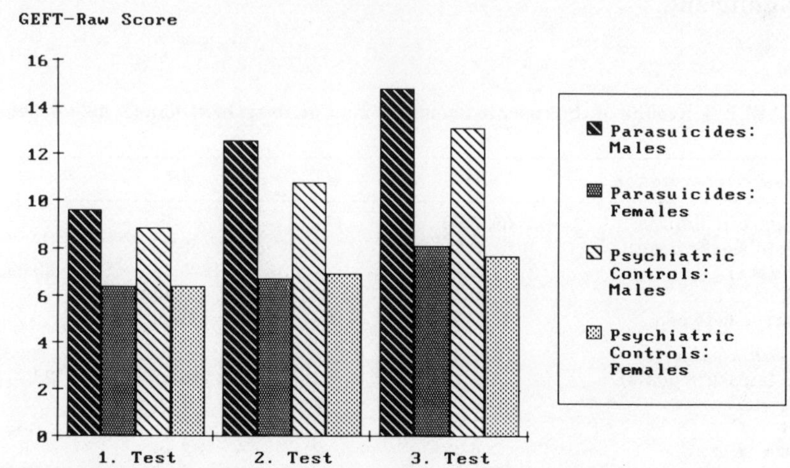

Figure 2: Field-dependence scores of tested groups over time.

TABLE 2: Results of analysis of variance: field dependence (including normal controls)

Source of variation	*SS*	*df*	*MS*	*F*	*Results of the a posteriori test*
A (classification)	1502.88	2	751.44	31.02	S/C, P/C
B (sex)	109.78	1	109.78	4.53	Sm/Cm, Sm/Cf, Sf/Cm, Sf/Cf
A × B	5.26	2	2.63	0.11	Pm/Cf, Pf/Cm, Pf/Cf, Cm/Cf
Error	6056.68	250	24.23		
Total	7674.59	255			

Tables 4 and 5 show the results obtained concerning dichotomous thinking. We found no differences between parasuicides and psychiatric controls. The mean value for the total of extreme answers and of positive extremes was slightly lower for the parasuicide group, but due to the great variance of these values, the effect was not significant. For the same reason, we found no significant differences between parasuicides and psychiatric controls for the first and third measurements. With regard to the concept 'colour white', the results revealed the same tendencies, but again, no significant differences between parasuicides and psychiatric controls were detectable. Only the value for neutral answers was higher at the third compared with the first measurements, but due to the great variance this effect was also not significant.

TABLE 3: Results of the repeated measurement analysis of variance: field dependence

Source of variation	*SS*	*df*	*MS*	*F*
Between subjects	6525.90	111		
A (classification)	39.22	1	39.22	
B (sex)	1725.38	1	1725.38	39.39
A × B	30.73	1	30.73	
Error between	4730.57	108	43.80	
Within subjects	2598.53	224		
C (measurements)	512.14	2	256.07	28.45
A × C	3.31	2	1.66	
B × C	131.81	2	65.91	7.32
A × B × C	6.32	2	3.16	
Error within	1944.95	216	9.00	

TABLE 4: Results of dichotomous thinking

Extremes	*Parasuicides*	*Psychiatric controls*
Total		
1. Test	35.18	35.09
3. Test	28.65	37.22
Positives		
1. Test	22.44	20.39
3. Test	16.59	23.34
Negatives		
1. Test	12.74	14.69
3. Test	12.06	13.97
Neutral		
1. Test	12.58	13.19
3. Test	13.92	14.22

TABLE 5: Results of dichotomous thinking: colour white

Extremes	*Parasuicides*	*Psychiatric controls*
Total		
1. Test	21.05	21.35
3. Test	19.24	25.65
Positives		
1. Test	19.45	19.11
3. Test	18.87	23.15
Negatives		
1. Test	1.60	2.40
3. Test	0.37	2.50
Neutral		
1. Test	39.87	31.82
3. Test	47.35	37.47

Discussion

Field dependence seems to be a common feature of all psychiatric patients. Observable differences between groups of parasuicides and psychiatric controls would, therefore, seem to reflect a general difference between the sexes with regard to this peculiar cognitive style, rather than differences between different diagnoses and suicidal behaviour as has been reported in previous studies (e.g., Levenson, 1972, 1974; Levenson and Neuringer, 1974). In crises, this cognitive style also seems to be more affected in men than in women. Therefore, the next step for research should be to test whether this effect is related to an absolute value: e.g. a higher degree of field independence, because the field-dependence values are age related (Panek, 1985), and men have higher mean values than women (Oltman *et al.*, 1971; Huss and Kayson, 1985).

It also seems probable that dichotomous thinking is a state rather than a trait variable. Our results further indicate that it is perhaps useless to try to measure dichotomous thinking by applying neutral concepts. Therefore, we conclude that dichotomous thinking is more linked with concepts of self-evaluation and may only be measurable during depressive states. The great range of variances in the findings for this variable also seems to reflect the existence of clusters of different persons or patients. Therefore, in further studies, we intend to analyse the influence of different person variables connected with this cognitive style and to perform cluster-analyses of patients with regard to these cognitive styles.

On the basis of our findings, we are unable to find grounds for support of the general hypothesis that suicidal patients are, as a whole, persons whose perception of their environment is undifferentiated, inarticulate, and global (Levenson, 1974). However, there may be a subgroup whose specific thinking style and cognitive characteristics can influence their interpretation and evaluation of potentially suicide-triggering circumstances—and the consequences of such behaviour—to such an extent that they are capable of only perceiving certain situations in one particular way. Being unable to recognise alternative solutions to such problems, their coping abilities are reduced so that only restricted and stereotyped solutions to problems are available to them (Levenson, 1972; Neuringer, 1964, 1974; Schrader *et al.*, 1986). This seems to be independent from the general intelligence score. Thus, suicidal behaviour is more likely to appear to them as a subjectively practical problem-solving strategy (Shneidman and Farberow, 1957; Levenson, 1974; Clum *et al.*, 1979; Patsiokas *et al.*, 1979; Schotte and Clum, 1982). These findings could probably be satisfactorily integrated into a comprehensive theoretical model for the explanation of suicidal behaviour.

References

Clum, G.A., Patsiokas, A.T. and Luscomb, R.L. (1979). 'Empirically based comprehensive treatment program for parasuicide', *Journal of Consulting and Clinical Psychology*, 47, 937–45.

Eastwood, M.R., Henderson, A.S. and Montgomery, I.M. (1972). 'Personality and parasuicide: Methodological problems', *Medical Journal of Australia*, 1, 170–5.

Eysenck, H.J. (1967). *The Biological Basis of Personality*, Springfield: Thomas.

Fine, B.J. (1972). 'Field-dependent introvert and neuroticism: Eysenck and Witkin united', *Psychological Reports*, 31, 939–56.

Huss, E.T. and Kayson, W.A. (1985). 'Effects of age and sex on speed of finding embedded figures', *Perceptual and Motor Skills*, 61, 591–4.

Lester, D. (1970). 'Attempts to predict suicidal risk using psychological tests', *Psychological Bulletin*, 74, 1–17.

Levenson, M. (1972). 'Cognitive and Perceptual Factors in Suicidal Individuals', dissertation, University of Kansas.

—— (1974). 'Cognitive correlates of suicidal risk', in C. Neuringer (ed.), *Psychological Assessment of Suicidal Risk*, Springfield: Thomas, 150–63.

—— and Neuringer, C. (1971). 'Problem-solving behaviour in suicidal adolescents', *Journal of Consulting and Clinical Psychology*, 37, 433–6.

—— (1974). 'Suicide and field dependency', *Omega*, 5, 181–6.

Megargee, E.L. (1967). 'Undercontrolled and overcontrolled personality types in extreme antisocial aggression', *Psychological Monographs*, 80 (3)(whole no. 611).

—— Cook, P.E. and Mendelsohn, G.A. (1967). 'Development and validation of an MMPI scale of assaultiveness in overcontrolled individuals', *Journal of Abnormal Psychology*, 72, 519–28.

Neuringer, C. (1961). 'Dichotomous evaluations in suicidal individuals', *Journal of Consulting Psychology*, 25 (5), 445–9.

—— (1964). 'Rigid thinking in suicidal individuals', *Journal of Consulting Psychology*, 28 (1), 54–8.

—— (1967). 'The cognitive organization of meaning in suicidal individuals', *Journal of General Psychology*, 76, 91–100.

—— (1974). 'Validation of the cognitive aspect of Adler's theory of suicide', *Journal of Individual Psychology*, 30, 59–64.

—— and Lettieri, D.J. (1982). *Suicidal Women: Their Thinking and Feeling Patterns*, New York: Gardner Press.

Oltman, P.K., Raskin, E. and Witkin, H.A. (1971). 'The Group embedded Figures Test: GEFT', Palo Alto: Consulting Psychologists Press.

Orbach, I. and Glaubman, H. (1978). 'Suicidal, aggressive, and normal children's perception of personal and impersonal death', *Journal of Clinical Psychology*, 34, 850–7.

Panek, P.E. (1985). 'Age differences in field-dependence/independence', *Experimental Ageing Research*, 11 (2), 97–9.

Parkes, K.R. (1981). 'Field dependence and the differentiation of affective states', *British Journal of Psychiatry*, 139, 52–8.

Patsiokas, A.T., Clum, G.A. and Luscomb, R.L. (1979). 'Cognitive characteristics of suicide attempters', *Journal of Consulting and Clinical Psychology*, 47, 478–84.

Raven, J.C. (1971). 'Standard Progressive Matrices. 2. Aufl.', London: Lewis & Co. Ltd.

Rothe, E. (1980). 'Beispiele für Suizidversuche bei Heranwachsenden. Bedrängt von Elternhaus und Schule', *Krankenpfleger Journal*, 18, 11–28.

Schmidtke, A. & Schaller, S. (1987). 'WITKIN-EFT Gruppentest'. Weinheim: Beltz.

Schotte, D.E. and Clum, G.A. (1982). 'Suicide ideation in a college population: A test of a model', *Journal of Consulting and Clinical Psychology*, 50, 690–6.

Schrader, G., Gibbs, A. and Harcourt, R. (1986). 'Dysfunctional attitudes

in former psychiatric inpatients', *Journal of Nervous and Mental Disease*, 174 (11), 660–3.
Shneidman, E.S. and Farberow, N.L. (1957). 'Clues to suidice', in E.S. Shneidman and N.L. Farberow (eds), *Clues to Suicide*, New York: McGraw-Hill, pp. 3–10.
Smith, E.J. (1981). 'Adolescent suicide—A growing problem for the school and family', *Urban Education*, 16, 279–96.
Spiegel, D.E. and Neuringer, C. (1963). 'Role of dread in suicidal behavior', *Journal of Abnormal and Social Psychology*, 66, 507–11.
Wetzel, R.D. (1975). 'Suicide intent, affect and cognitive style', *Dissertation Abstracts International*, 36 (6B), 3080.
Williams, J.M.G. and Broadbent, K. (1986). 'Autobiographic memory in suicide attempters', *Journal of Abnormal Psychology*, 95 (2), 144–9.
Witkin, H.A., Oltman, P.K., Raskin, E. and Karp, S.A. (1971). *A Manual for the Embedded Figures Tests*, Palo Alto, Calif.: Consulting Psychologists Press.
Witkin, H.A. and Goodenough, D.R. (1977). 'Cognitive styles: Essence and origins. Field dependence and field independence', Psychological Issues, monograph 51, New York: International Universities Press.
—— and Oltman, P.K. (1979). 'Psychological differentiation: Current status', *Journal of Personality and Social Psychology*, 37, 1127–45.

Suicide and aggression: a comparison of autoaggressive and externally aggressive persons in the Nuremberg municipal area

T.A. MOESLER and W. WEIDENHAMMER

Introduction

In 1940 Germany, the great psychiatrist Hans-Walter Gruhle (Gruhle, 1940) pointed out the connection between suicide actions and externally aggressive bodily injuries. He also suspected relationships in the geographical distribution of autoaggressive and externally aggressive persons or actions which could be analysed in ecological and socio-demographic terms.

So far, only a few researchers have compared autoaggressive and externally aggressive persons (Ferreira de Castro *et al.* 1986; Keltikangas-Järvinen, 1978; Modestin, 1986; Moesler *et al.* 1988) and even fewer have investigated the distribution of these groups of individuals in specific urban districts (Bagley *et al.* 1973; Moschel *et al.* 1981; Porterfield, 1952). Most recent studies focused on a comparison of persons after suicide actions with victims of violent crime. These investigations are based on the concept that the victims of external aggression have contributed to the violent act by an autoaggressive attitude 'being at the wrong place at the wrong time' (Holinger *et al.* 1987). Whatever one may think about this idea, clear correlations are to be found in the analysis of these two groups. Our study cannot provide any appraisal on victims of violent crime. However, we have some comparative results on autoaggressive and externally aggressive persons using data which have been collected in the context of a broad research project at our clinic. The focal point is the determination of environmental factors which might have promoted or impeded the autoaggressive and externally aggressive behavior of Nuremberg citizens.

This study has not yet been completed. For the present, we can only report preliminary results on the following criteria: age and sex distribution, marital status, unemployment, nationality, and domicile distribution over the city areas.

Methods

Within the period 1976–85, the files of 1143 persons who had committed suicide were evaluated in the City Health Office of Nuremberg. From 1979 to 1985, the patient records of 2583 persons after attempted suicide in the Nuremberg Municipal Hospital were also evaluated; altogether data were collected on 3726 autoaggressive persons.

The Police files of the Central Franconian Police Headquarters served for registering seventy-three externally aggressive perpetrators with fatal consequences and 10 573 perpetrators who had committed bodily injuries without fatal consequences. Because of the small number of perpetrators in the first group we did not include them in the analysis.

Table 1 shows the five most frequent types of aggressive criminal offences in Nuremberg. The criterion for external aggression was the threat of bodily harm or body contact. Insults and material damage, which some authors (Selg, 1986) also rate as externally aggressive, were not included.

In the specified period all autoaggressive and externally aggressive persons were registered who had become so abnormal in their actions that they appeared to require treatment in the opinion of their social environment, or the attention of the authorities had been drawn to them. Exclusively persons resident in Nuremberg were included in the study. Each person was included only once with their last autoaggressive or externally aggressive action. Thus, the results are person- not action-based. Of course, we are aware of undetected cases, the percentage of which is very

TABLE 1: Breakdown of aggressive criminal offences

The most frequent offences	*Percentage*
1. Mild intentional bodily injury	48
2. Grievous bodily harm	43
3. Robbery in general	2
4. Armed robbery	2
5. Rape	1

Note: The calculations are based on the statistics of crime of the police of Mittelfranken. The data include information about 10 573 perpetrators with aggressive criminal offences resident in Nuremberg in the years 1976–85.

difficult to estimate. However, this is not likely to have had crucial effects on our results. The focal point of our analysis was the comparative description of three groups: persons after suicide, persons after attempted suicide, and externally aggressive persons without fatal consequences.

Results

Some background information on the City of Nuremberg is given in Table 2.

The mean suicide rate (1976–85) was 23.4 per 100 000, somewhat higher than in West Germany, for which Schmidtke and Häfner (1985) calculated a rate of 21.3 in 1983. The overall ratio of suicide to attempted suicide and external aggression was about 1 to 3 to 9 in Nuremberg.

In Nuremberg there is a relatively low rate of attempted suicide compared with suicide. Even if a high percentage of cases has gone undetected, and considering the fact that we only recorded the last attempted suicide for each individual, this must be rated as a special feature of the Nuremberg population for which we still do not have a satisfactory explanation.

As expected, most suicides and the highest incidence of external aggression was found in men. Women made about twice as many attempts at suicide and only about 15 per cent of the externally aggressive actions of the men (Table 3).

In the age-specific distribution of aggressive actions the rating applies to externally aggressive persons. Besides the relatively high aggression in youth and early adulthood, the relatively high external aggression of the 26–45-year-old women is striking. Overall, women are about half as frequently externally aggressive

TABLE 2: Nuremberg population statistics (mean results for the years 1976–85)

	Male		*Female*
	%	%	%
Total population: 483 887	46.3		53.7
Age: < 25 years	29.3		25.2
25–65 years	58.8		53.4
> 65 years	11.9		21.4
Percentage of foreigners	12.7		9.2
Religion			
Protestant		47.9	
Catholic		36.1	
None		11.6	

TABLE 3: Rates for persons with suicide, parasuicide and aggressive criminal offences (without death), averaged for the years 1976–85 (parasuicide 1979–85), Nuremberg (per 100 000 inhabitants)

		Mean annual suicide rate	*Mean annual parasuicide rate*	*Mean annual aggressive offence rate*
Total population	483 887	23.4	75.7	218.5
Male	224 061	29.2	50.7	398.2
Female	259 826	18.4	97.2	63.6

as autoaggressive. On the other hand, men are, on average, five times as frequently externally aggressive as autoaggressive. There appears to be a two-peak curve for male suicide, with a fall in the 46–60 years age group. After the age 26–45 years externally aggressive actions decrease whilst successful suicide increases. With greater age, the aggression is self-directed.

This general distribution pattern of autoaggressive and externally aggressive behaviour was equally pronounced in comparable analyses of other researchers (Keltikangas-Järvinen, 1978; Moesler *et al.* 1988). This indicates that age- and sex-specific relations essentially mask life-phase and regional influences.

The marital status breakdown of our three groups compared with the overall population is given in Table 4. We disaggregated by age, because of the relationship between marital status and age. For further interpretation we focused on the age group 26–60 years. Statistical testing was not carried out on the other age groups because sample sizes were too small to achieve reliable results.

Unmarried men as well as divorced and widowed persons of both sexes show a tendency to successful suicide compared with the overall population. The percentages of single men and divorced persons of both sexes as well as of widowed men are higher within the group of attempted suicide. Mainly unmarried men and divorced persons of both sexes showed externally aggressive behaviour. Without exception marriage appeared to be of protective significance with regard to autoaggressive and externally aggressive behaviour.

In a more detailed analysis of autoaggressive persons aged over sixty (Moesler *et al.* 1988), it was shown that widowed men had the highest risk of dying from suicide or making an attempted suicide, followed by unmarried men. In women of this age group divorced

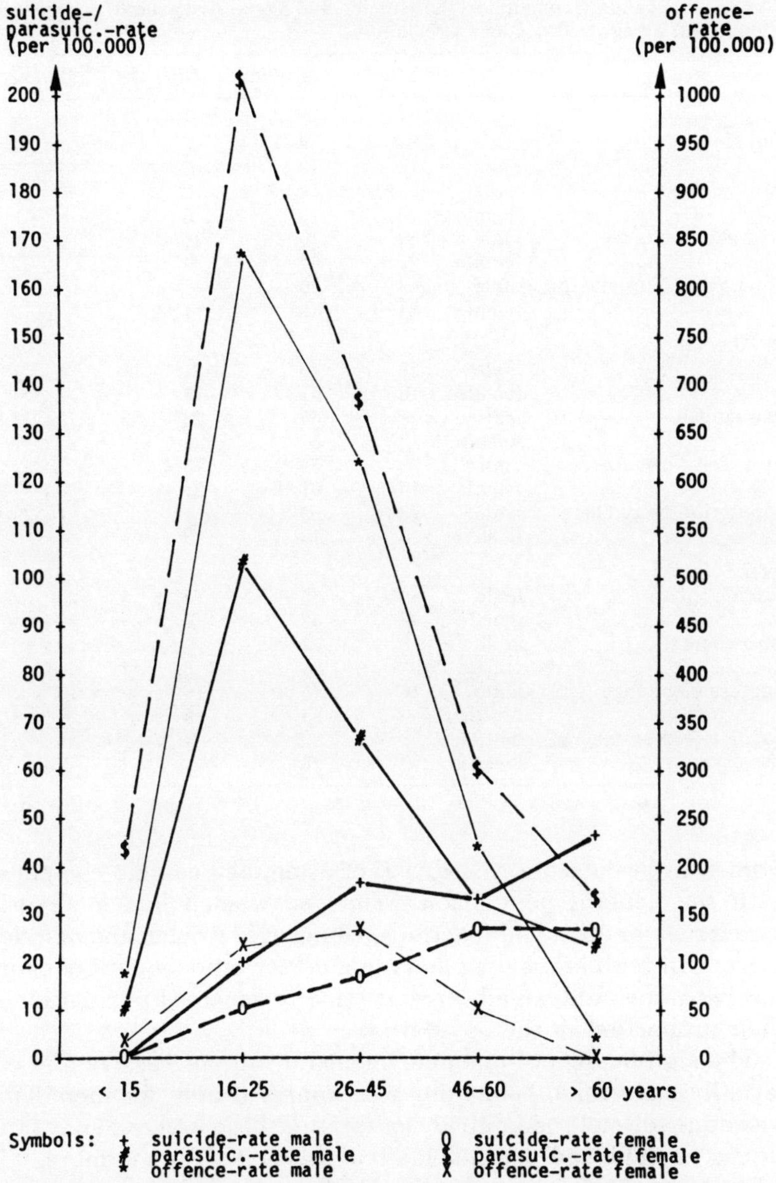

Figure 1: Age- and sex-specific rates for persons with suicide, parasuicide, and aggressive criminal offences in Nuremberg, 1976–85 (per 100 000 inhabitants per year)

TABLE 4: Breakdown of suicide, parasuicide and aggressive groups, and general population, by age and gender (percentages)

		Single	*Married*	*Divorced*	*Widowed*
15–25 years					
Suicide	male	88	9	3	–
	female	79	19	2	–
Parasuicide	male	85	13	2	–
	female	79	15	6	–
Aggressive offence	male	89	10	1	–
	female	62	34	4	–
Population Nuremberg	male	93	6	–	–
	female	84	15	1	–
26–60 years					
Suicide	male	27	49	21	3 (**)
	female	16	51	19	13 (**)
Parasuicide	male	27	49	22	2 (**)
	female	13	56	28	4 (**)
Aggressive offence	male	26	58	15	1 (**)
	female	15	61	21	3 (**)
Population Nuremberg	male	23	69	7	1
	female	16	70	10	4
Over 60 years					
Suicide	male	4	65	3	28
	female	9	32	7	52
Parasuicide	male	3	52	5	40
	female	4	34	8	54
Aggressive offence	male	6	68	15	10
	female	–	65	9	26
Population Nuremberg	male	3	80	4	13
	female	9	35	7	49

(**): $p < 0.01$

women experienced a raised risk of attempted suicide compared with the general population. Widowed women had a slightly raised risk for all suicidal actions. Unmarried women and married persons of both sexes over sixty committed suicide actions more rarely than would have been statistically expected in relation to their proportion in the population.

The significance of unemployment for autoaggressive and externally aggressive behaviour was analysed only for men. This was done for methodological reasons since the assignment of the status 'unemployed' is problematical in women. Furthermore, it is difficult to obtain a standardised definition of that status since different databases have to be compared.

In the population of Nuremberg the unemployment rate among men was 3.1 per cent. In the suicide group we found a rate of 5.3 per cent and in the attempted suicide group a rate of 17.3 per cent.

TABLE 5: Percentages of foreigners within the groups 'suicide', 'parasuicide', and 'aggressive offence', compared to the total population of Nuremberg

Foreigners	*Male*	*Female*
	%	%
Suicide	2.9 (**)	1.7 (**)
Parasuicide	7.7 (**)	10.9 (*)
Aggressive offence	27.1 (**)	25.9 (**)
Population Nuremberg	12.7	9.2

(*): $p < 0.05$; (**): $p < 0.01$

The externally aggressive men showed the highest rate of unemployment (30.7 per cent). Thus, unemployment was shown to be an important factor both for autoaggressive and externally aggressive behaviour.

The proportion of foreigners in our three groups differed from the overall population (Table 5). Foreigners have a significantly lower risk of suicide. In attempted suicide a slightly raised risk was found for foreign women,but a lowered risk for men. In externally aggressive persons we found a markedly increased rate both in male and female foreigners.

We determined the domicile for all autoaggressive and externally aggressive persons. We then analysed the residential areas of Nuremberg with a high and a low incidence of the three forms of aggression. On the basis of the variables available to us it was shown that the characteristics deviating least from the average could be found for districts with a high proportion of successful suicides. This indicates that, to a certain degree, the occurrence of suicide is independent of the environment. The greatest deviations in the analysed variables were shown in districts with many externally aggressive persons, whereas the districts with many attempted suicides were in the middle (Table 6).

A high percentage of divorced persons was characteristic for all districts with an extreme incidence of aggressive behaviour whereas surprisingly, the proportion of Catholics did not affect the extreme groups.

Conclusion

Three prototypes for the residential areas concerning autoaggressive and externally aggressive persons can be constructed in Nuremberg from the variables available to us.

(*1*) The typical residential area with a high suicide rate shows

TABLE 6: Description of districts with extreme rates for persons with suicide, parasuicide and aggressive criminal offences (lowest vs highest 20 per cent of the distribution)

Variable	*Suicide*		*Parasuicide*		*Aggress. offences*	
	↓	↑	↓	↑	↓	↑
Number of inhabitants	− −	+ +			+ +	− −
Percentage of						
old people	− −	+ +				
children > 6 yrs			−	+	+	−
women 15 − 25 yrs					− −	+ +
divorced	− −	+ +	− −	+ +	− −	+ +
single					− −	+ +
Number of births (German)			− −	+ +	−	+
Percentage of						
foreigners			− −	+ +	− −	+ +
Protestants			+ +	− −	+ +	− −
Catholics						
without confession			−	+	− −	+ +
Inhabitants per hectare			− −	+ +		
Mobility			− −	+ +	− −	+ +
Percentage of						
living space					+ +	− −
commercial space					− −	+ +
post-war buildings					+ +	− −
apartments without bathroom					− −	+ +
Density of rest./bars					− −	+ +
Density of motor vehicles					+ +	− −
Percentage of cars with high cubic capacity					− −	+ +

−/+ : decreased/increased ($p < 0.05$)
− −/+ +: decreased/increased ($p < 0.01$)

a great number of inhabitants, a high percentage of elderly persons as well as divorced persons.

(*2*) The highest risk of attempted suicide is found in a district with a high percentage of divorced persons, high birth rate, high percentage of foreigners, low percentage of Protestants, high residential density, and high mobility.

(*3*) Characteristic for externally aggressive persons is a district with the following features: small number of inhabitants, high percentage of 15–25-year-old women, high percentage of divorced or single persons, high percentage of foreigners, high mobility, little living area, a large proportion of industrial area, many public houses or bars, many flats without bathroom which were built before 1948, and many cars with large engines.

This paper is limited to a description of the residential environment where the highest rates of suicide, attempted suicide, and externally aggressive behaviour are to be expected. The questions of which people show suicidal or aggressive behaviour, and whether there is a relationship with environmental factors will be answered in further analysis.

References

Bagley, C., Solomon, J. and Palmer, C. (1973). 'Social Structure and the Ecological Distribution of Mental Illness, Suicide and Delinquency', *Psychological Medicine*, 3, 177–87.

Ferreira de Castro, E., Albino, L. and Martins, I. (1986). 'Suicide and Homicide in Portugal', *Acta psychiatrica Scandinavica*, 74, 425–32.

Gruhle, H. (1940). 'Geographie des Selbstmords', *Der Nervenarzt*, 8, 337–41.

Holinger, P.C., Offer, D. and Ostrov, E. (1987). 'Suicide and Homicide in the United States: An Epidemiologic Study of Violent Death, Population Changes and the Potential for Prediction', *American Journal of Psychiatry*, 144, 215–19.

Keltikangas-Järvinen, L. (1978). 'Personality of Violent Offenders and Suicidal Individuals', *Psychiatria Fennica*, 57–63.

Modestin, J. (1986). 'Über die Beziehung zwischen Kriminalität und Suizidalität', *Fortschritte der Neurologie, Psychiatrie*, 54, 289–96.

Moesler, T.A., Welz, R. Weidenhammer, W. and Demling, J. (1988). 'Suizidhandlungen des höheren Lebensalters im Nürnberger Stadtgebiet von 1976 bis 1985', in K. Böhme and E. Lungershausen (eds.), *Suizid und Depression im Alter*, Regensburg: Roderer.

Moschel, G. Häberle, H. and Welz, R. (1981). 'Zur innerstädtischen Verteilung sozialer Devianz in Mannheim', in H. Walther (ed.), *Region und Sozialisation*, vol. 1, Stuttgart: Frommann und Holzboog.

Porterfield, A.L. (1952). 'Suicide and Crime in the Social Structure of an Urban Setting: Fort Worth, 1930–1950', *American Sociological Review*, 17, 341–9.

Schmidtke, A. and Häfner, H. (1985). 'Suicide und Suicidversuche': Epidemiologie in der Bundesrepublik Deutschland', *Münchener Medizinische*

Wochenschrift, 127, 828–32.
Selg, H. (1986). Personal remark.

Acknowledgements

We are indebted to the Nuremberg Health Department, the President of the Franconian Police Department, and the clinical directors of the Municipal Hospital at Nuremberg: Prof. Dr Dieter Platt, 2nd Department of Internal Medicine and University Institute of Gerontology; Prof. Dr Walter Pontzen, Department of Psychosomatics; and Dr Manfred Fleischmann, Department of Neurology. Furthermore, we thank Dr Trutzel and Mr Schneider of the Amt Für Stadtforschung at Nuremberg for their friendly advice.

Suicide attempters' attitudes towards short-term treatment on a psychiatric ward of a university hospital

A.P. VISSER and A.J.F.M. KERKHOF

Introduction

The number of suicides in the Netherlands has doubled since 1950. The number of suicide attempts also increased markedly, so that over the past fifteen years the number of hospital admissions after suicide attempts has nearly doubled. At a rough estimate, annually more than 25 000 suicide attempts are medically treated in Dutch hospitals (Diekstra *et al.* 1982; Gezondheidsraad, 1986). From two studies among hospital staff it can be concluded that while there are set procedures to provide psychiatric care during hospital stay, the liason with mental health care often does not function very well (Kerkhof *et al.* 1983; Kerkhof *et al.* 1988). These conclusions are supported by the results of a study carried out among Dutch suicide attempters about their experience with treatment in a general hospital and with subsequent mental health care (Kerkhof, 1985). It is stressed that management policy does not meet sufficiently the needs of suicide attempters, who want their problems to be taken seriously and to be given emotional support, a need which the nursing staff does not always recognise. Suicide attempters also mentioned distrust and anticipation of blame and punishment. Consequently, any open communication with those who were treating them was impeded. There are also indications that those who have attempted suicide in the past receive less attention from medical staff. The research findings link up with conclusions noted elsewhere about professional care for suicide attempters (Hawton and Catalan, 1982; Platt and Salter, 1987; Reimer, 1983).

It can be concluded that mental health care has not always been successful in preventing suicide attempters from repetition.

Improvement in suicide prevention may be found in the better management of those treated in hospital because of the physical consequences of a suicide attempt. In this respect, information about the attitudes of suicide attempters about their treatment in hospitals is an important opportunity to improve the therapeutic ward climate. Feedback to psychiatrists, nursing staff, and social workers on the quality of treatment of patients was shown to be a forceful means to bring about adequate care delivery (Visser, 1988). An important factor related to this is that data about the attitude of patients should be measured in a reliable and valid way.

In this chapter we describe the results of a study about the tuning of short-term treatment to the needs of suicide attempters at the psychiatric ward of the University Hospital of Leiden. At the request of the ward staff, an inquiry has been set up among patients about their attitudes to their hospital stay and the perceived patient-centered ward climate. They filled out a questionnaire which was discussed with the nurses. In this way information about the attitudes of patients was available to the staff, and so there was an opportunity to reduce identified care problems. The following points were important in the inquiry among patients.

In the first place the study was not only confined to the group of suicide attempters but, for comparative reasons, data were also collected among patients who had been admitted for other reasons. This design offers the possibility of drawing conclusions about (*a*) the relative seriousness of complaints of suicide attempters about their treatment; and (*b*) the extent to which the feedback procedure contributed to the perceived patient–staff interaction.

Secondly, the study relied on experience acquired with a validated and standardised way of measuring hospital patients' attitude (Visser, 1988). The latter concept is interpreted as multidimensional, in which a distinction has been made between satisfaction, emotional state, and perceived patient-centered ward climate. Satisfaction refers to the extent to which patients judge (positively or negatively) the nature of treatment as they experienced it on the ward. Important aspects of the emotional state of patients are: acceptance of the admission, stress experienced at time of admission and later on during their stay, and the perception of openness to personal problems. The perceived patient-centered ward climate refers to the extent to which attention is paid to emotional support, learning to deal with problems, and the perceived professionality of the staff. Research among patients in general hospitals shows that patients who judge the patient-centered climate more favourable are also more satisfied on various points about the treatment received. At the same time, a more favourable emotional state is positively related to a higher satisfaction with treatment (Visser, 1988).

A third point about the survey was the assumption that the attitude of patients is influenced by individual characteristics of patients. In particular, younger patients often judge the hospital stay more negatively than elderly patients (Kerkhof, 1985; Visser, 1988).

Research based on these three points should result in a more specific insight into the nature of the attitude of the hospital treatment of suicide attempters, which could be relevant for improving the care for this group of patients. To summarise: the study is directed towards answering the following questions:

(*1*) To what extent do suicide attempters' attitudes towards short-term treatment differ from those who have been admitted to the psychiatric ward for other reasons?

(*2*) Is there a relationship between treatment satisfaction, emotional state and the perceived patient-centered ward climate among suicide attempters?

(*3*) To what extent are suicide attempters' attitudes towards hospital stay affected by age, sex, length of stay in hospital, and type of referral to subsequent health care?

Method

Altogether, 199 patients took part in the survey. They had been admitted during the years 1985, 1986, and 1987 to the psychiatric ward of the University Hospital of Leiden. In the course of 1985 the old accommodation, consisting of four provisionally separated beds in one room, was replaced by nine new, individual patient rooms. The nursing staff asked the patients to participate in the survey in which they were requested to discuss on the day of their discharge relevant points of the questionnaire they had completed. Patients completed the questionnaire independently on the eve of their discharge. They submitted the completed questionnaire to one of the nurses. All patients were eligible for the survey; only occasionally was a questionnaire not completed. The necessary biographical information about the patients, in-

TABLE 1: Measured concepts and questions asked (number)

Satisfaction
Quality of the treatment with regard to attention paid to problems during treatment (3)
Contribution to the treatment (sympathy of, contact with and time available of: psychiatrist (3), nurses (3), social workers (3)
Stay in general: atmosphere, meals, and privacy (3)
General satisfaction: patient wants to be admitted there again in future, recommend ward to friends (2)
Emotional state
Acceptance of stay at admission and later on during stay, felt at ease, proper length of stay (4)
Stress (uncertainty, being ill at ease, anxiety, distrust) at admission and later on (2)
To be able, to want, and to dare to discuss personal problems (3)
Ward climate
Emotional support received (2)
Professional and open attitude of staff members (4)
Having been taught to deal with problems, usefulness of stay (2)

cluding whether a suicide attempt had been made, was obtained in 1987 from administrative files. In some cases, this information was missing.

The questionnaire consisted of two sections. The first section included sixteen 'satisfaction' questions allowing patients to rate from 1 (= low) to 10 (Visser, 1988). Questions concerned the following: quality of dealing with problems in general; contribution of doctors, nurses and social workers in terms of showing sympathy; nature of the contact and the time available; and questions about the stay in general (atmosphere, meals, privacy), and the way friends and relatives were taken care of. The second part of the questionnaire consisted of questions with various response alternatives dealing with: satisfaction with the nursing department in general; being able to make complaints; the emotional state and its acceptance at the admission; attentiveness to personal problems; emotional support and help received; judging of the duration of the admission; and contacts with fellow patients.

Based on the results of a factor analysis and the intended meaning of the questions, internally consistent measures have been developed (Table 1). The mean alpha-coefficient for the several concepts is 0.72 (range 0.49–0.89).

Results

Table 2 contains information about some background characteristics of the patients, with a comparison between suicide attempters and patients admitted for other reasons. It shows that the total group of patients mainly consists of female patients; the main age group is 41–60 years; the average length of stay is 8.1 days, whereas most patients (61 per cent) stay at the ward for less than one week. After their stay, half of the group of patients had been referred to the outpatients' clinic of the hospital. The longer the stay, the more the patients are referred to a general psychiatric hospital. Comparison between both groups of patients shows that those who attempted suicide are significantly younger and stay on the ward for a short period of time than patients who have been

TABLE 2: Background characteristics of suicide attempters and patients admitted for other reasons

Background characteristics	*Total group of patients*	*Suicide attempters (Max N = 66)*	*Other reason admission (Max N = 85)*
Age (N = 151)			
Younger than 30 years	21.8	22.1	14.1
30–40 years	17.9	22.7	14.1
41–60 years	40.4	38.8	49.4
Older than 60 years	19.9	16.7	22.4
Average age	43.9 yrs	40.3 yrs*	46.8 yrs*
Sex (N = 152)			
a. Male	31.6	31.8	30.6
b. Female	68.4	68.2	69.4
Length of admission (N = 149)			
2–3 days	22.1	29.2	16.7
5–7 days	38.9	44.6	34.5
8–13 days	28.2	18.5	35.7
Longer than 2 weeks	10.7	7.7	13.1
Average length in days	8.1	6.9*	9.0*
Referral to (N = 148)			
Outpatient clinic	50.4	46.9	53.7
Community mental health centre and other out-patient treatment	25.2	29.7	21.9
Psychiatric hospital	11.6	14.1	9.8
Remainder, no referral	12.2	9.4	14.6
Location (N = 199)			
Old accommodation	15.1	24.2	16.5
New accommodation	84.9	75.8	83.5

*T-tests; $p \leqslant 0.02$; chi-square-tests $p \leqslant 0.04$; two-tailed tests. (Number of respondents may vary because of missing data)

admitted for other reasons. In the presentation of data about the attitude of both groups, the difference in age and length of stay is taken into account.

Satisfaction

The results indicate that, generally speaking, patients awarded relatively high marks to various aspects of their stay on the ward. More than 10 per cent of the patients give a low score (1–5) to: the amount of time made available by the social worker (18.2 per cent), the appreciation of the contact with the social workers (13.5 per cent), the extent to which treatment is successful in dealing with the problem (12.8 per cent), sympathy of the social worker for their problems (10.9 per cent), appreciation of contacts with the nursing staff (10.8 per cent), and the atmosphere in general (10.1 per cent). It seems that help supplied by the social worker was judged least favourably (see also the average scores shown in Table 3). There were no significant differences in satisfaction between suicide attempters and those who were admitted for other reasons, even after taking into account differences in age and length of stay between these two groups (covariance analysis).

Generally speaking, patients appeared to be relatively satisfied with various aspects of their stay. The average satisfaction scores differ little from those of patients from general hospitals (see Table 3) with the exception of aspects concerning their stay in general, which are valued higher in the general hospital. In reply to the question concerning whether topics about which they were dissatisfied could be discussed with the staff, 74.9 per cent of the patients answered affirmatively; 16.4 per cent replied 'not everything', and 8.7 per cent answered negatively. Table 3 shows that the more patients thought that their criticism was open for discussion, the more satisfied they were on various aspects of their stay. The mean correlation for suicide attempters is only a little lower in comparison with the other group ($r = 0.24$ and 0.32, respectively). Differences between the groups are most marked with regard to judgement of the quality of treatment in general, satisfaction with the nursing staff, and general satisfaction. For suicide attempters, criticism on these points seemed more difficult to discuss than for other groups of patients.

The results indicate that, in reaching a qualified treatment, it is important that there is an open atmosphere at the nursing departments, enabling patients to discuss their complaints.

TABLE 3: Satisfaction of the patients

Aspects of satisfaction	*Total group*		*Hospital patients*[a]	*Suicide attempters*	*Other patients*	*Correlation with possibility to discuss complaints*	
						Suicide attempters	*Others*
	$\bar{x}$	*s.d.*	$\bar{x}$	$\bar{x}$	$\bar{x}$	$\bar{x}$	$\bar{x}$
Quality of treatment with regard to attentiveness to problems	7.8	1.5	(7.3)	7.9	7.8	0.17	0.47***
Contribution to the treatment (sympathy, contact, time) by:							
psychiatrist	7.7	1.6	(7.7)	7.6	7.9	0.31**	0.34**
nursing staff	8.2	1.3	(8.1)	8.2	8.3	0.23*	0.39***
social worker	7.5	2.0	(7.6)	7.6	7.5	0.14	0.18
Stay in general: atmosphere, meals, privacy	8.2	1.3	(7.8)	8.1	8.3	0.30**	0.15
Taking care of friends and relatives	8.2	1.6	(na)	8.1	8.4	0.18*	0.22*
General satisfaction	7.8	1.4	(7.6)	7.7	7.8	0.33**	0.51***

*$p \leqslant 0.05$; **$p \leqslant 0.01$; ***$p \leqslant 0.001$; Pearson correlation coefficients; one-tailed tests; na: not available.
[a]Derived from Visser (1988)

Emotional state and ward climate

The results shown in Table 4 indicate that patient groups do not differ in their judgement of their emotional state and the perception of the ward climate. This holds true even after controlling for differences in age and length of stay. Most patients have a positive judgement of their emotional state and the ward climate. Some examples are:

—agreement to admission (average of questions 88.5 per cent);

—stress at admission (56.0 per cent), but not later on (73.3 per cent);

—86.1 per cent of the patients discussed their personal problems with staff-members;

—not having received emotional support (an average of 9.3 per cent);

—professional and open attitude of the staff (88.5 per cent);

—the admission has a positive significance with regard to the problems (an average of 88.9 per cent).

The correlations in Table 4 indicate that usually a positive relationship exists between the emotional state and the perceived ward climate, except for the experience of stress at admission and later on. There are few differences in correlations between groups of patients. However, it appears that there is a stronger relationship between the patient-centered ward climate and the extent to which problems are discussed among suicide attempters. For the non-suicide attempters there seems a stronger relationship between acceptance of admission and the extent to which these patients appreciate the ward climate.

The general conclusion is that a favourable perceived ward climate benefits the emotional state of the patients. This also applies to patients who have been admitted on account of a suicide attempt.

Satisfaction, emotional state, and ward climate

Table 5 describes the relationship between the indices of satisfaction and data about their emotional state and perceived ward climate. The correlations indicate that, generally speaking, for both groups of patients there was a positive association between satisfaction with emotional state and perceived ward climate. One exception is the relationship with stress experienced at admission and afterwards. Among non-suicide attempters, there was a weak correlation between satisfaction with the social worker and emotional state. We have already seen that patients direct most of

TABLE 4: Emotional state and perceived ward climate

Indicators of emotional state and ward climate	*Total group* $\bar{x}$	*s.d.*	*Suicide attempters* $\bar{x}$	*Other patients* $\bar{x}$	*Correlation between emotional state and ward climate*[a] *sa*	*nsa*
Emotional state						
Acceptance of hospital stay	12.7	2.2	12.8	12.7	0.22*	0.31***
Stress experienced	4.4	1.3	4.5	4.3	−0.10	−0.06
Discussion of personal problems	8.9	1.9	9.0	8.9	0.40***	0.24*
Ward climate						
Emotional support received	6.8	0.8	6.8	6.9		
Professional and open attitude of staff	3.6	0.7	3.5	3.7		
Having been taught to deal with problems	5.7	1.4	6.0	5.6		

*p ⩽ 0.05; **p ⩽ 0.01; ***p ⩽ 0.001; Mean Pearson correlation for ward climate indices
[a]sa = suicide attempters; nsa = non suicide attempters

TABLE 5: Relation of indices of satisfaction, emotional situation, and ward climate

	Quality of treatment		*Psychiatrist*		*Nurses*		*Social worker*		*Atmosphere*		*In general*	
	sa	*nsa*	*sa*	*nsa*	*sa*	*nsa*	*sa*	*nsa*	*sa*	*nsa*	*sa*	*nsa*
Emotional state[a]												
Acceptance of admittance	0.60**	0.47**	0.24*	0.33**	0.51**	0.51**	0.28*	0.03	0.22*	0.06	0.49**	0.59**
Stress	−0.06	0.01	−0.09	−0.02	0.12	−0.14	−0.17	−0.16	0.20	−0.20*	−0.28**	−0.01
Discussion of personal problems	0.37**	0.24*	0.45**	0.17	0.34*	0.23*	0.38*	0.12	0.24*	0.22*	0.28**	0.37**
Ward climate	0.46**	0.55**	0.54**	0.55*	0.47**	0.46**	0.49**	0.28*	0.23*	0.35**	0.41**	0.47**

*$p \leqslant 0.05$; **$p \leqslant 0.01$; Pearson correlation coefficients; one tailed tests; for ward climate mean Pearson correlation coefficients.
[a]sa = suicide attempters; nsa = non suicide attempters

their criticism against the social worker, who appears more successful in satisfying the needs of suicide attempters than those who have been admitted for other reasons.

Changes during the investigation

The project continued for a period of three years. Taking into account the positive judgement of the ward climate by patients, the question arises whether the support of the patients has gradually improved on account of feedback supplied to the staff. In considering changes over time, possible differences arising from age and length of stay of the patients are taken into account, as are the interaction effects with patient group. Analyses of covariance show only main effects for the factor 'year of study'. The satisfaction with the doctor, support of relatives, a professional and open attitude of the staff, and having been taught to deal with problems is higher during the third year. It is suggested that there is a developing learning process on the part of the staff, and that, particularly in the third year of the study, improvements occurred in the perceived ward climate and patients' satisfaction.

Background characteristics

The correlations between independent variables are accounted for by age, length of stay, and sex of patients both for suicide attempters and non-suicide attempters. For the group of suicide attempters, it shows that older patients experienced a stronger general satisfaction (if necessary they would return and recommend the ward to friends) and indicates more strongly that they were able to discuss their personal problems ($r = 0.26$ and $r = 0.21$, respectively). Female suicide attempters are more critical about the ward climate. In the group of non-suicide attempters, older patients are more satisfied with the social worker ($r = 0.29$). In general, it can be concluded that personal background characteristics do not substantially influence the attitude towards short-term treatment on this psychiatric ward.

Discussion and conclusion

In a study among patients of the psychiatric ward of the University Hospital of Leiden, attitudes among patients admitted because of a suicide attempt were examined. In the survey, a distinction was made between three aspects of patients' attitude: satisfaction with various aspects of the stay; the emotional state of the patients; and the perceived climate at the ward concerning psychosocial care. A standardised and validated questionnaire was used, one which had been developed in research among patients in general hospitals (Visser, 1988). The group of suicide attempters was compared with a group of patients admitted for other reasons. It was found that between these two groups there were no significant differences regarding satisfaction, the emotional state, and the perceived ward climate. Significant associations were found between the three aspects of experience. The conclusion can be drawn that a more favourable ward climate goes together with a better emotional state and a higher level of patient satisfaction.

In view of the fact that individual factors like age, sex, length of stay, and kind of referral to the health care hardly affect the attitude of the patients, the conclusion seems justified that the nature of the support supplied has a particularly favourable contribution to the satisfaction of suicide attempters about their care. This result can be attributed to the practice developed by the nursing staff in the ward of discussing completed questionnaires with the patients. In this way information about the attitude of patients is available to the staff, and, in consultation, they try to solve the problems identified. In previous studies it was found that feedback about the experience of patients was an important means for improving patient care (Harris, 1978; Visser, 1988). This approach also seems an important factor in the treatment of suicide attempters, because hospitals perform an important role in the prevention of repetition of suicide attempts. The study described here shows that information about the attitude of the patients offers the possibility of tuning the policy concerning short-term psychosocial treatment more towards the needs of suicide attempters. The previously identified unfavourable attitude to suicide attempters (Kerkhof, 1985; Platt and Salter, 1987) can be improved by means of feedback to health workers about the experiences of patients.

In this study, patients had been informed beforehand that the completed questionnaire would be discussed with them on the day of their discharge. The question arises whether this approach led to more favourable answers. However, we think this is unlikely. We would like to point out that studies among patients in general hospitals show that a more anonymous way of interviewing by means of a written survey does not produce results which differ from those obtained orally (Visser, 1988). We would also like to point to the conclusion of Bergsma (1976) that improvement of the patient-centered climate went together with a more realistic patient attitude. A personal interview with patients at the hospital reinforced the social desirability tendency, leading to more favourable answers (Visser *et al.* 1988).

Further studies on the evaluation of care for suicide attempters might give an indication about the possible influence of the way of interviewing by varying anonymity and paying attention to the influence of the social desirability factor on the answering of the questions. Improving the method of interviewing patients would thus contribute to improving the quality of care delivered to attempted suicide patients, and possibly to the prevention of repetition.

References

Bergsma, J. (1976). 'Evaluatie van een kommunikatieprojekt in een algemeen ziekenhuis', *Mens en Ondern*, 30, 5–22.

Diekstra, R.F.W., de Graaf, A.C. and van Egmond, M. (1982). 'Over de epidemiologie van suicidepogingen', *Tijdschrift voor Sociale Geneeskunde*, 20, 398–404.

Gezondheidsraad (1986). *Advies inzake suicide*, Rijswijk.

Harris, R.T. (1978). 'Improving Patient Satisfaction through Action Research', *Applied Behavioural Science*, 14, 382–99.

Hawton, K. and Catalan, J. (1982). *Attempted Suicide*, Oxford: Oxford University Press.

Kerkhof, A.J.F.M., Moritz, B.J.M., Maliepaard, R.A. and Diekstra, R.F.W. (1983). 'Het beleid in de Nederlandse ziekenhuizen t.a.v. niet-somatische aspecten van opvang, behandeling en verwijzing van suicidepogers', *Tijdschrift voor Sociale Gezondheidszorg*, 61, 938–44.

Kerkhof, A. (1985). *Suicide en de geestelijke gezondheidszorg*, Lisse: Swets en Zeitlinger.

Kerkhof, A.J.F.M., Wiegers, T., Silvester, C. and Waenink, P. (1988). *Hulpverlening na suicidepogingen*, Leiden: D.S.W.O. press.

Platt, S. and Salter, D. (1987). 'A comparative Investigation of Health Workers' Attitudes towards Parasuicide', *Social Psychiatry*, 222, 202–8.

Reimer, C. (1983). 'Problems of interaction with suicidals', in J.P. Soubrier and J. Vedrinne (eds.), *Depression and Suicide*, Paris/London: Pergamon Press.

Visser, A.Ph. (ed.)(1988). *Onderzoek naar de tevredenheid van ziekenhuispatiënten: doel methode en beleid*, Lochem/Gent: De Tijdstroom.

——, Breemhaar, B. and Kleijnen, J.G.V.M. (1988). *The Role of Social Desirability in Program Evaluation in Health Care*, paper at the 1st European Conference on Programme Evaluation, Leiden: 16/17 The Netherlands.

Acknowledgement

We are greatly indebted to the staff and the patients of the ward for their contribution to the survey, particularly to Karin van Brussel.

The prognostic value of hopelessness in patients following a suicide attempt

T. DIETZFELBINGER, A. KURZ, A. TORHORST and H.J. MÖLLER

Introduction

The results of different studies describing hopelessness or pessimism as an essential characteristic of depression with a special relation to suicidality (Beck, 1963) induced Beck *et al.* (1974) to develop the 'Hopelessness Scale', an instrument designed to determine hopelessness in a standardised manner. In the following years, as a result of further studies, several authors drew the conclusion that hopelessness could be the connecting link between depression and suicide (Minkoff *et al.* 1973; Beck *et al.* 1975; Wetzel, 1976; Dyer and Kreitman, 1984).

It is a question not only of theoretical but also of practical interest whether the Hopelessness Scale has a predictive value with respect to relapse of suicidal behaviour. For this purpose, Beck *et al.* (1985), in a prospective study, examined more than 200 patients with present suicidal ideation who had not made a recent suicide attempt. After more than five years, they compared the data of the persons who had died from suicide in the meantime with the data of the remaining patients, and found significantly higher values on the Hopelessness Scale in the first group. How many more patients had attempted suicide during the follow-up period without dying and what degree of hopelessness this group had were not examined.

In the present study, the German version of the Hopelessness Scale (Krampen, 1979) was used on a large sample of patients who had recently attempted suicide. The first aspect we analysed was the relationship between the Hopelessness Scale, actual psychopathological state and personality traits. The second aspect was the predictive value of the Hopelessness Scale with respect to parasuicidal relapse and other dimensions over a one-year follow-up period.

Method

The sample comprises 247 non-psychotic patients who were admitted to the Toxicology Department of the Technical University Hospital in Munich for in-patient detoxification following a suicide attempt. Compared with the total population of Munich, the following subgroups were over-represented: persons under forty years of age, singles, divorced, and unemployed persons. These socio-demographic data are largely in agreement with the data presented in two earlier studies concerning suicidal patients in Munich (Kockott *et al.* 1970; Möller *et al.* 1978).

The diagnoses were made in accordance with the ninth Revision of the ICD. In all 28 per cent of the patients had a neurosis, 11 per cent had a personality disorder, 44 per cent suffered from a reactive disorder, 15 per cent were classified with the primary diagnosis 'abuse/dependence', and 2 per cent with 'others'. For approximately three-quarters of the patients this was their first suicide attempt; one-quarter of them admitted one or several suicide attempts in the past. The first examination of the patients was carried out as soon as possible after in-patient admission, the follow-up one year later.

Besides the Hopelessness Scale, following instruments were used (Table 1):

One factor (*Anxious Depression* (*ANX*)) *of the IMPS* (Lorr, 1974), an internationally used observer rating scale for psychopathology;

The Global Assessment Scale (*GAS*)(Endicott *et al.* 1976), with

TABLE 1: Data sources at the time of the index examination and at a 1-year follow-up

Index Examination	*1-year follow-up*
ANX (IMPS)	ANX (IMPS)
GAS	GAS
D-S	D-S
FPI	FPI
HS	
CL	
	Recurrence of parasuicide (yes/no)

which the examiner globally assesses aspects of psychopathology and disturbances in social adjustment;

The Depressivity Scale (*DS*), comprising present depressive tendencies, and the *Complaint List* (*CL*), containing discomfort. The standardised Self-Rating Scales were both developed by von Zerssen (1976);

The Freiburg Personality Inventory (*FPI*)(Fahrenberg *et al.* 1978), often used in German-speaking areas. This questionnaire describes pre-morbid personality on the basis of the patient's self-evaluation. It comprises nine standard scales ascertained by factor analysis as well as the three item-analytically constructed supplementary scales.

The Hopelessness Scale and the Complaint List had been presented to the patients during the index examination whereas all other instruments were provided when starting the study and at one-year follow-up. Moreover, recurrence of parasuicide within one year subsequent to the index examination was monitored.

In order to investigate the relationship between hopelessness and personality traits and actual psychopathological state, Pearson correlation coefficients were calculated between the Hopelessness Scale and all other factors of the instruments used at the time of index examination. Additionally a secondary factor analysis was calculated over all eighteen factors.

The predictive value of the Hopelessness Scale was determined by calculating the correlation between the Hopelessness Scale and the following outcome criteria: Global functioning (GAS), observer-rated depressivity (ANX of IMPS), and self-evaluated depressivity (D-S) at one-year follow-up, as well as recurrence of parasuicide within one year.

Correlations between hopelessness, actual psychopathological state and personality traits

The Hopelessness Scale correlates significantly with both observer rating-scales (Table 2) used, a little higher with the ANX-scale of the IMPS ($r = 0.35$, $p < 0.001$) than with the GAS ($r - -0.23$, $p < 0.01$), which represents more generally the level of functioning. Evidently higher and also significant are the correlation coefficients between the two self-evaluation scales developed by von Zerssen and the Hopelessness Scale (Table 3): $r = 0.51$ ($p < 0.001$) with the Depressivity Scale and $r = 0.47$ ($p < 0.01$) with the Complaint List. In Table 4 correlation coef-

TABLE 2: Correlations between the Hopelessness Scale and observer rating-scales

	Hopelessness Scale	
Anxious Depression (IMPS)	0.35	$p < 0.001$
Global Functioning (GAS)	−0.23	$p < 0.01$

ficients between the Hopelessness Scale and the twelve dimensions of the Freiberg Personality Inventory (FPI) are listed. The correlation coefficient of 0.59 between the FPI dimension 'depressiveness' and the Hopelessness Scale is especially remarkable. We should point out that this factor refers to a depressive personality characteristic and not the present depressive symptoms, as it is the case in the Depressivity Scale by von Zerssen.

In a secondary-factor analysis over all eighteen factors used (Table 5) we decided on a three-factor solution because of content, as well as for statistical reasons (Scree-Test according to Cattell). The Hopelessness Scale formed a common factor with the ANX-factor of the IMPS, with both self-evaluation scales by von Zerssen concerning depressivity and physical complaints, as well as the FPI dimensions nervousness and (negative) masculinity. The factor analysis thus shows a closer relation of the Hopelessness Scale towards depressivity as a symptom, as it is shown in the ANX scale or the Depressivity Scale by von Zerssen, and less relation to the personality-oriented depressivity aspects as it is expressed in the FPI-scale depressivity. This dimension, however, forms, together with other factors of the FPI the secondary factor 2, whereas the further five FPI dimensions form the secondary factor 3. To this, the following note should be made: the FPI handbook states the result of a factor analysis which was only calculated with the twelve FPI dimensions; the two factors which form a two-factor solution largely correspond in their combina-

TABLE 3: Correlations between the Hopelessness Scale and v. Zerssen's self-evaluation questionnaires (D-S and CL)

	Hopelessness Scale	
Depressivity Scale	0.51	$p < 0.001$
Complaint List	0.47	$p < 0.01$

TABLE 4: Correlations between the Hopelessness Scale and the Freiburg Personality Inventory (FPI)

			Pearson correlation (r) with the Hopelessness Scale	
FPI	1	Nervousness	0.48	$p < 0.001$
FPI	2	Spontaneous aggressivity	0.29	$p < 0.001$
FPI	3	Depressiveness	0.59	$p < 0.001$
FPI	4	Excitability	0.30	$p < 0.001$
FPI	5	Sociability	0.43	$p < 0.001$
FPI	6	Stability	−0.40	$p < 0.001$
FPI	7	Reactive aggressivity/ dominance striving	0.22	$p < 0.01$
FPI	8	Inhibition	0.48	$p < 0.001$
FPI	9	Frankness	0.12	ns
FPI	E	Extroversion	−0.25	$p < 0.01$
FPI	N	Neuroticism	0.47	$p < 0.001$
FPI	M	Masculinity	−0.51	$p < 0.001$

tion with the secondary factors 2 and 3 of the factor analysis in the present study.

On the whole it can be determined that the Hopelessness Scale has a closer relation to depressivity at the level of symptoms than to depressivity at the level of personality; moreover, the examined personality dimensions show a typical relation among themselves.

The predictive value of the Hopelessness Scale

The correlations between the Hopelessness Scale at the time of index examinations and the different outcome criteria are listed

TABLE 5: Secondary-factor analysis (three-factor-solution)

Factor 1:	*Hopelessness Scale* Anxious Depression (IMPS) Complaint List Depressivity Scale FPI 1 Nervousness FPI M Masculinity (negative)
Factor 2:	FPI 4 Excitability FPI 2 Spontaneous aggressivity FPI 7 Reactive aggressivity FPI 9 Frankness FPI N Neuroticism
Factor 3:	*5 other FPI-dimensions*

TABLE 6: Correlations between the Hopelessness Scale and outcome criteria

	Hopelessness at the time of index estimation	
Anxious depression (IMPS) at follow up	0.24	$p < 0.01$
Global functioning (GAS) at follow-up	−0.17	ns
Self-evaluated depressivity (D-S) at follow-up	0.29	$p < 0.001$
Recurrence of parasuicide at follow-up	0.13	ns

in Table 6. The association with anxious depression is low but significant, whereas the association with the GAS is not significant. The correlation coefficient between the Hopelessness Scale and the recurrence of parasuicide within one year is only 0.13 and is not statistically significant. During the follow-up period of one year twenty-five patients attempted suicide once or several times, i.e. approximately 10 per cent of the initial sample.

Another six patients died of suicide during this follow-up period. It was not possible to analyse the predictive value of the Hopelessness Scale with respect to eventual suicide on the basis of this small group. Therefore, a comparison of the results of the present study with the data from Beck *et al.* (1985) cannot be made.

Summary

In a multi-dimensional assessment, Beck's Hopelessness Scale was correlated fairly highly with depressivity. A correlation analysis and a secondary-factor analysis demonstrated a closer relationship between the Hopelessness Scale and actual depressive symptoms than depressivity as a personality trait. The value of the Hopelessness Scale as a predictor of one-year outcome was rather low, expecially with respect to recurrence of parasuicide during the follow-up period.

References

Beck, A.T. (1963). 'Thinking and Depression', *Archives of General Psychiatry*, 9, 324–33.

——, Weissman, A., Lester, D. and Trexler, L. (1974). 'The Measurement of Pessimism: The Hopelessness Scale' *Journal of Consulting and Clinical Psychology*, 42, 861–5.

Beck, A.T., Kovacs, M. and Weissman, A. (1975). 'Hopelessness and Suicidal Behavior: An Overview'. *Journal of the American Medical Association*, 234, 1146–9.

Beck, A.T., Steer, R.A., Kovacs, M. and Garrison, B. (1985). 'Hopelessness and Eventual Suicide: A 10-year Prospective Study of Patients

Hospitalized with Suicidal Ideation', *American Journal of Psychiatry*, 142, 559–63.

Dyer, J.A.T. and Kreitman, N. (1984).'Hopelessness Depression and Suicidal Intent in Parasuicide', *British Journal of Psychiatry*, 144, 127–33.

Endicott, J., Spitzer, R.L., Fleiss, J.L. and Cohen, J. (1976). 'The Global Assessment Scale: A Procedure for Measuring Overall Severity of Psychiatric Disturbance', *Archives of General Psychiatry*, 33, 766–71.

Fahrenberg, J., Selg, H. and Hampel, R. (1978). *Das Freiburger Persönlichkeitsinventar FPI*, Hogrefe.

Kockott, G., Heyse, H. and Feuerlein, W. (1970). 'Der Selbstmordversuch durch Intoxikation', *Fortschritte der Neurologie Psychiatrie*, 38, 441–56.

Krampen, G. (1979). 'Hoffnungslosigkeit bei stationären Patienten—Ihre Messung durch einen Kurzfragebogen (H-Skala)', *Z. Med. Psychol.*, 5, 39–49.

Lorr, M. (1974). 'Assessing Psychotic Behavior by the IMPS', in P. Pichot (ed.), *Psychological Measurements in Psychopharmacology, Modern Problems of Pharmacopsychiatry* (Basel), Vol. 7, Paris: Karger.

Minkoff, K., Bergman, E. and Beck, R. (1973). 'Hopelessness, Depression, and Attempted Suicide', *American Journal of Psychiatry*, 130, 455–9.

Möller, H.J., Werner, V. and Feuerlein, W. (1978). 'Beschreibung von 150 Patienten mit Selbstmordversuch durch Tabletten unter besonderer Berücksichtigung des Selbstmordverhaltens und der Inanspruchnahme von Beratungsmöglichkeiten für Suizidgefährdete', *Archiv fuer Psychiatrie und Nerrenkrankheïten*, 226, 113–35.

Wetzel, R.D. (1976). 'Hopelessness, Depression, and Suicide Intent', *Archives of General Psychiatry*, 33, 1069–73.

Zerssen, D.v., unter Mitarbeit von Koeller, D.M. (1976). 'Klinische Selbstbeurteilungs-Skalen (KSb-S) aus dem Münchner Psychiatrischen Informationssystem (PSYCHIS München), Manuale: a) allgemeiner Teil, b) Paranoid-Depressivitäts-Skala, c) Befindlichkeits-Skala, d) Beschwerden-Liste. Beltz, Weinheim.

Attempted suicide by jumping from a height: a five-year retrospective study

X. POMMEREAU, P. TEDO and F. PENOUIL

In France, jumping from a height is the method used by 4 per cent of male and 10 per cent of female suicide completers (Davidson and Philippe, 1986). In England and Wales, we observe the same rate among male completers but only 5 per cent among female completers (McClure, 1987). However, among women, the rate of suicide mortality by jumping has risen by 67 per cent during the period 1975–84 (Table 1).

On the other hand, attempted suicide by jumping from a height is a rare event concerning, on average, only one or two suicide attempters out of 100 (Table 2). Despite the spectacular nature of this method and its emotional impact on the general population, the fact that it is a rare event probably explains both the small

TABLE 1: Numbers (and rates per million population) for suicide by jumping from a high place (E 957) in England and Wales, 1975–84(*)

	1975		*1984*		
	Number	*Rate*	*Number*	*Rate*	*Change in rate 1975–84*
Female	*46*	*1.8*	*77*	*3.0*	+ *67*
Male	*110*	*4.6*	*144*	*4.7*	+ *2*

(*) Data from McClure (1987)

TABLE 2: Frequency percentage rate of jumping among suicide attempters

Source	*Number of patients*	*Percentage jumping*
		%
Davidson and Philippe (1986), 1980–Lyon, Bas-Rhin	*3 273*	*1.1 (male)* *1.3 (female)*
Garros et al. *(1988), 1986–Aquitaine*	*5 000*	*2*

number of studies focused on this method and the reduced size of the samples studied (Prasad and Lloyd, 1983).

Material and method

Located in a catchment area of 640 000 inhabitants, the Bordeaux University Medical Centre deals with 2000 suicidal cases each year, of which 95 per cent involve self-poisoning (especially drug overdose), and 3–4 per cent involve a violent method (five out of ten of these by firearms, three out of ten by jumping from a height, and two out of 10 by cutting or piercing). The annual number of suicide attempters by jumping who were still alive and referred to our hospital represents one-fourth of the total number of hospitalised persons using this method in the region of Aquitaine.

The present work is a retrospective study of people who survived an attempted suicide by jumping and who were admitted to our hospital during a five-year period from 1 January 1982 to 31 December 1986 (in all some 110 patients). Thirty eight were male, seventy-two female; none was under fifteen years of age. For each patient, we consulted the medical file of admission and summarised the nature of medical and surgical care administered, outcome and follow-up, including out-patient treatment. Most patients (96 per cent) had been evaluated by a psychiatrist during their hospitalisation: 65 per cent by the psychiatrist of the unit, the remainder by another psychiatrist. Every general practitioner involved was contacted by letter to obtain additional information: the response was 75.5 per cent. Of patients who were alive eight days after the attempt, 26 per cent were reviewed by the psychiatrist of the unit within a period of one to three years after the attempt.

Table 3 shows that the mortality rate at the eighth day among

TABLE 3: Mortality rate at the eighth day among 1982–6 sample and suicide attempters, by jumping, in Aquitaine, 1986

	Mortality at the eighth day	
Jumping from a Height	*n*	*%*
1982–6 sample (N = 110)	22*	20.0
Aquitaine, 1986 (N = 92)	19	20.8

*Seven males; fifteen females

TABLE 4: Severity of physical damage and middle-term mortality among suicide attempters, by jumping, after eighth day

	Male (N = 31)		*Female (N = 57)*	
	n	%	*n*	%
Low severity*	18	58.0	28	49.0
Medium severity**	11	35.5	22	38.5
High severity***	2	6.5	7	12.5
1982–6 mortality in relation to the original act	2	6.5	4	7.0

*Lenth of stay in surgical ward less than forty-five days; no or minimal residual handicap
**Length of stay in surgical ward forty-five days to four months; orthopaedic residual handicap
***Tetraplegia, hemiplegia with or without other associated residual handicap

our sample was 20 per cent (18 per cent among males, 21 per cent among females), similar to the rate in Aquitaine (21 per cent).

Table 4 indicates the degree of physical damage in relation to the length of stay in surgical wards and the nature of residual handicap. These data lack the systematic precision of the Injury Severity Score (ISS), but the latter was not always used in Bordeaux during the study period. Nevertheless, it appears that the physical state of the patients is more relevant to evaluation than the distance fallen, which is often measured subjectively.

Obviously, jumping from a height causes multiple lesions. In our sample, we observed 39 per cent with cranial lesions, 54.4 per cent with vertebral lesions, 55 per cent with peripherical lesions, 29 per cent with abdomino-pelvic lesions, and 25.5 per cent with thoracic lesions. It is to be noted that these lesions were not specific to gender. The middle-term mortality rate among subjects living at the eighth day was 7 per cent.

Socio-demographic data

In Table 5, we compare two samples: suicide attempters by jumping, and by drug overdose. We observe a similar distribution in both groups according to sex and age. As far as those who attempted to commit suicide by jumping are concerned, we may note a socio-demographic 'profile': 70 per cent are under forty-five years old, two-thirds of the patients are females; single and inactive people predominate.

Psychiatric data

First of all, it is important to take into consideration that one

TABLE 5: Socio-demographic data comparing suicide attempters by jumping (1982–6) with suicide attempters by drug overdose referred to the same hospital in 1985–6

	Jumping (N = 110)		*Drug overdose (N = 3378)*	
	n	%	*n*	%
Age (in years)				
15–24	24	22 } 70%	953	28 } 80%
25–34	33	30	1 059	31
35–44	20	18	700	21
45–54	8	7	319	9.5
55 and over	25	23	296	9
Males	38	34.5	1 088	32
Females	72	65.5	2 290	68
Single	49	44.5	1 047	31
Married couple	40	36.5	1 486	44
Divorced/separated	10	9	743	22
Widowed	11	10	102	3
Unemployed males	2	5	675	20
Unemployed females	8	11	439	13
Economically active	67	61	1 114	33

male out of two (N = 19 patients) and one female out of four (N = 20 patients) had taken alcohol, pills, or drugs before jumping, possibly as disinhibiting factors.

In Tables 6(a and b) we again compare our sample with a representative group of suicide attempters by drug overdose. If the percentage of patients who had a history of previous suicide

TABLE 6a: Psychiatric data comparing suicide attempters by jumping (1982–6) with a representative group of suicide attempters by drug overdose (N = 908) referred to the same hospital in 1986

	Jumping (N = 110)		*Drug overdose (N = 908)*	
History	*n*	%	*n*	%
Previous suicide attempt	42	38	432	47.5
Previous psychiatric in-patient treatment	41	37	171	19
Psychiatric out-patient* treatment	40	36	191	21
Psychiatric in-patient* treatment	38	34.5	37	4
No psychiatric care*	29	26.5	662	73
Unknown	3	3	18	2

*At the time of the suicidal act

TABLE 6b: Psychiatric data comparing suicide attempters by jumping (1982–6) with a representative group of suicide attempters by drug overdose (N = 908) referred to the same hospital in 1986

Psychiatric diagnosis		*Jumping (N = 110)* *n*	*%*	*Drug overdose (N = 908)* *n*	*%*
Psychosis	M	11	29	31	11
	F	29	41	69	11
Neurosis	M	1	2.5	58	21
	F	22	30	164	26
Reactive disorder	M	2	5	97	35
	F	15	20	252	40
Borderline	M	6	15.5	50	18
	F	2	2.5	64	10
Alcoholism/addiction	M	7	18	33	12
	F	4	5	44	7
Undetermined or other	–	11	10	46	5

attempts appears to be smaller among our sample (38 per cent) than among drug overdosers (47.5 per cent), it must be noted that eight out of every ten suicide attempters by jumping who had this antecedent had made at least one previous attempt by drug overdose.

Most suicide attempters by jumping had a psychiatric history and one-third of the patients (34.5 per cent) committed their suicidal act during in-patient treatment (nine out of ten in a psychiatric institution).

Psychiatric diognoses are shown in Table 6b: among our sample, 29 per cent of males, 41 per cent of females were psychotic (including schizophrenic and affective forms). Female patients with a diagnosis of neurotic disorder were assessed as hysterical/histrionic in nine cases out of ten. In both sexes, we observe a small number of reactive disorders. Finally, the proportion of

TABLE 7: Percentage of patients who later complete/re-attempt suicide, 1982–7, among sample (N = 82)

	Male (N = 29) *n*	*%*	*Female (N = 53)* *n*	*%*
Completed suicide*	1	3	1	2
Suicide attempt* (at least 1)	3	10	6	11
Unknown	5	17	4	7.5

*Jumping was re-used in nine cases out of eleven

patients with mental illness reached 64.5 per cent in our sample, compared with 56.5 per cent among the drug overdose attempters.

The repetition rate in our sample, from 1982 to 1987, is shown in Table 7: we may note that 10 per cent of the patients had made another suicidal attempt, of which 2 per cent were fatal, during the study period: jumping from a height was the method used again in nine out of eleven cases.

Discussion

Most of the suicide attempters by jumping from a height are young, female, economically inactive, and suffering from a psychiatric illness. More than one-third committed their suicidal act as psychiatric in-patients.

The socio-demographic characteristics found in our sample differ radically from those described by Kontaxakis *et al.* (1988) in a smaller group (N = 46) of suicide attempters by jumping referred to the Out-patient Department of Athens University: these patients were more often men, of a more advanced age, close to characteristics observed among suicide completers. These Greek data seem to reflect a local specificity because jumping from a height appears to be the most frequently used method of suicide in the Greek urban population (Beratis, 1986).

On the other hand, our findings agree with the fact that jumping from a height usually indicates serious psychiatric disorder, in particular psychosis (Sims and O'Brien, 1979; Prasad and Lloyd, 1983; Kontaxakis *et al.* 1988). In Table 8, we show the rate of psychosis among four different sample groups of suicide attempters in France, and observe that this rate is higher in our sample (three times higher for males, four to seven times higher for females).

It is also not surprising to note a lower rate of reactive disorders among suicide attempters by jumping compared with those who used drug overdose (see Table 6b). It is probably more surprising at first glance to observe both the young age of the subjects and the sex-related frequency of hysteria (with a prevalent female rate) among jumpers of our sample.

In fact, whatever the nature of the psychiatric disorders considered (whether psychosis or hysteria), a number of common phenomenological traits can be found with great frequency, for example:

—there is an absence of premeditation, the action being com-

TABLE 8: Psychosis rate among four samples of suicide attempters

	Male		*Female*	
	Total sample	*% Psychosis*	*Total sample*	*% Psychosis*
Jumping 1982–6 (Bordeaux–France) N = 110	38	29	72	41
Drug overdose 1986 (Bordeaux–France) N = 908	277	11	631	11
Attempted suicide 1980* (Lyon–France) N = 2122	697	10.6	1425	6.5
Attempted suicide 1980* (Bas Rhin–France) N = 1151	390	9.2	761	5.9

*Data from Davidson and Philippe (1986): nine suicide attempters out of ten used drug overdose

mitted on a sudden impulse;

—a peculiar atmosphere seems to prevail at the time the action is committed. This resembles a depersonalisation experience, a 'casting-off' gesture of a truly symbolic nature, and is often induced or enhanced by the simultaneous absorption of disinhibiting drugs (alcohol, psychotropics, psychodysleptics. . .);

—there is a concept of a 'complete' act, of a 'true' act, in which the subject propels his entire body from the inside out, thus giving (more than by any other method of suicide) reality to the notion of 'crossing over', and, therefore, of 'transgression'.

From a metapsychological viewpoint, Freud (1920) approached this field of jumping from a height via its symbolically representative contents (the fall), by looking at the case of a young lesbian women who jumped from a bridge, uttering the now classic formula 'NiederKommen'. If the interpretation given by Freud is, by nature, difficult to use outside its context, nevertheless, phenomenological traits appear in his observations which are similar to those described above, namely sudden impulse, constraint, and depersonalisation. We may also note the importance of the look of the eyes, 'everything being played in the twinkling of an eye'. This fundamentally scopic aspect places the attempted suicide by jumping in the area of the 'specular', apparently reflecting a set of radically narcissistic problems. For it was indeed from the rapturous enjoyment of his own image that Narcissus could not tear himself away, his fascination proving to be lethal. If it can be admitted that this method of suicide specifically calls into question the problem of the other self, as we hypothesise in Figure 1, then this model of narcissistic failure could become the object of a more thorough psychopathological study.

Conclusion

A relatively rare, but often devastating, suicidal act, jumping from a height is a method which reaches a high dramatic intensity, particularly due to the impulsive nature of the act and the 'spectacular' form it usually takes.

Our study confirms that this method of suicide is more often perpetrated by females; people who use this method most often suffer from a severe mental pathological disease, unlike those who attempt suicide by drug overdose. But what seems to us most worthy of note is the frequency with which many 'jumpers' describe a depersonalisation experience in the moments before

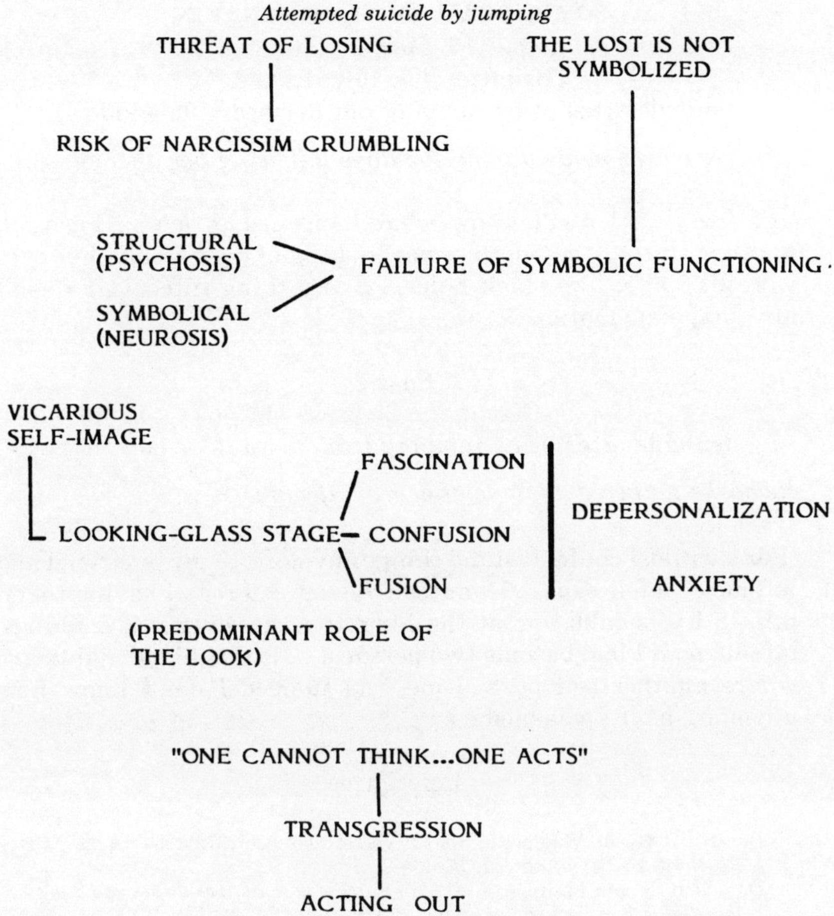

Figure 1: Model of narcissistic failure

their action. This characteristic leads us to hypothesise that this particular method of suicide is linked to a set of radically narcissistic problems, and that it poses the question, more so than any other suicidal method, of the basic relation of the subject to his or her other self.

Case 1

Brigitte . . . , 16 years old
(suicide attempt by jumping out her bedroom window)

Remarks made during the days following her attempt:

'It's fuzzy. . . I don't know what happened to me. . . I was in another state. . . my mother was looking at me harshly, her eyes were like pits, like black holes. . Every thing tilted. . . I wasn't any shape anymore. . .'

Case 2

Gisèle. . . , 27 years old
(suicide attempt by jumping from a 3rd floor balcony)

Remarks gathered 15 days after her attempt:

'For a while, I couldn't stand things anymore. . . my boyfriend had left me. . . I felt bad. . . I wanted to sleep. . . I recall having taken pills. . .I was calm and at the same time nervous. . . I could see myself, as if I had become two persons. . . It was like a nightmare where another self pushed me. . . I jumped I don't know how anymore, as if I was pushed. . .'

References

Beratis, S. (1986). 'Suicide in South Western Greece 1979–1984', *Acta Psychiatrica Scandinavica*, 74, 433–9.

Davidson, F. and Philippe, A. (1986). *Suicide et tentatives de suicide aujourd'hui: étude épidémiologique*, Paris: INSERM/DOIN.

Freud, S. (1920). 'Sur la psychogénèse d'un cas d'homosexualité féminine', *Névrose, Psychose et Perversion*, 1973, Paris: PUF.

Garros, B. *et al.* (1988). 'Accidents et intoxications en Aquitaine', Enquéte INSERM/ORSA, in press.

Kontaxakis, V. *et al.* (1988). 'Attempted Suicide by Jumping: Clinical and Social Features', *Acta Psychiatrica Scandinavica*, 77, 435–7.

McClure, G.M.G. (1987). 'Suicide in England and Wales, 1975–1984', *British Journal of Psychiatry*, 150, 309–314.

Prasad, A. and Lloyd, G.G. (1983). 'Attempted Suicide by Jumping', *Acta Psychiatrica Scandinavica*, 68, 394–6.

Sims, A. and O'Brien, K. (1979). 'Autokabalesis: An Account of Mentally Ill People who Jump from Buildings', *Medicine, Science and the Law*, 19, 195–8.

5

CLINICAL MANAGEMENT AND AFTERCARE OF PARASUICIDE

Compliance

H.J. MÖLLER

The problem of compliance is currently being considered more frequently and more thoroughly in the fields of medical care and psychotherapy; in the latter regard, this problem appears to be of special interest in the area of suicide prevention (Kurz and Möller, 1984).

Compliance and its background factors

From research work in psychotherapy and drug therapy we know some relevant background factors affecting compliance (Graupe, 1975; Linden, 1979). Based on these results we should keep in mind that compliance with therapy is a very complex phenomenon, constituted mainly by the triangle of patient, therapist, and therapy. In addition, institutional and other aspects have to be considered. With respect to the patient, the following variables, among others, seem to be relevant: social class, personality traits, insight into illness or problems, whether suffering from illness, information about therapy, expectations about therapy, experiences during the therapeutic sessions, and experiences from former psychotherapy. As to the therapist: social class, personality traits, theoretical background, type and duration of psychotherapeutic education, duration of working as psychotherapist, etc., are of importance.

Based on clinical evidence, it can be concluded that suicidal patients, especially those who have just attempted suicide, can be characterised as an unfavourable group with respect to some factors relevant for compliance. Often they show unstable and/or narcissistic personalities, problems in establishing interpersonal relationships, a lack of insight into their disturbance, a low degree of suffering from their problems, little information about psychotherapy, and a weak interest in psychotherapy. Many of them prefer to complain about their emotional trouble or to manipulate their partners with suicide gestures or attempts rather than to work seriously on changing their own situation.

However, the unsatisfying compliance rates cannot be related only to these patient characteristics; other aspects are also of great relevance, as will be demonstrated in the following presentation of our own findings.

Non-compliance as a problem of suicide prevention

As already mentioned, compliance rates in suicide prevention as recorded in the literature are generally low (Kurz and Möller, 1984). With respect to treatment in suicidal crises, the compliance can be estimated to be about 50 per cent (Table 1). The compliance with treatment following parasuicide seems to be still lower, about 30–40 per cent if compliance-related procedures have not been performed. This might be at least partially explained by two facts:

(*a*) many of these patients after parasuicide do not come by their own motivation but are referred by a physician;

(*b*) the parasuicide itself and the change in environmental conditions brought about by the parasuicide reduce the motivation for therapy.

Our own experiences were gathered mostly with parasuicide patients of two large hospitals in Munich: the Krankenhaus München-Schwabing and the Klinikum rechts der Isar. Nearly all these patients under investigation were admitted to the hospital because of self-induced intoxication. The samples investigated are very similar with respect to social and psychiatric background data representing the typical clientele of parasuicide patients of

TABLE 1: Compliance in suicidal crises and after parasuicide

Compliance in suicidal crises	%	*Compliance after parasuicide*	%
Hankoff and Walter (1968)	33	Bogard (1970)	11
Murphy *et al.* (1969)	50	Paykel *et al.* (1974)	45
Slaiken *et al.* (1977)	46	Oast and Zitrin (1974)	26
Sudak *et al.* (1977)	63	Morgan *et al.* (1976)	70
		Häfner (1978)	44
		Hankoff *et al.* (1979)	34

primary compliance	30 - 40 % of parasuicide patients
remaining in therapy >2 hours	~ 60 % of Arche patients
effective compliance	~ 24 % of parasuicide patients

Figure 1: Calculation of effective compliance under standard care conditions for parasuicide patients

general hospitals: predominantly younger people, women being over-represented, and a high percentage of patients with non-psychotic disturbances.

In general, the non-psychotic patients were, after detoxification and a short crisis intervention during their hospital stay, referred to the 'Arche', a special out-patient institution for suicide prevention and after-care in Munich.

In our first pilot study on compliance (Möller *et al.* 1978), we had the astonishing result that only ten of thirty-two patients being judged as motivated for after-care arrived at the 'Arche', a primary compliance rate of about 30 per cent (Figure 1). Based on a general drop-out rate (less than three sessions) of 40 per cent among the general 'Arche' clientele, we calculated an effective compliance rate of only 24 per cent (Möller *et al.*, 1978).

Fixed after-care arrangement as compliance factor

A first glance at the data of this pilot study led to the conclusion that patients for whom a fixed after-care appointment was arranged seemed to demonstrate greater compliance. This correlated with findings in the literature that parasuicide patients need special efforts to bring them to therapy (Kurz and Möller, 1985). This hypothesis seems to be meaningful in the context of the above-mentioned fact that parasuicide patients are not positively selected with respect to motivation, personal stability and other factors relevant for compliance.

We tried to test this hypothesis in another sample (Möller and Geiger, 1981), in which a fixed after-care appointment was arranged as often as possible, an approach which was limited only by the capacity of the 'Arche'. For 77 percent of 132 patients such an appointment could be reached. The general compliance rate was increased from 31 per cent in the earlier study to 55 per cent

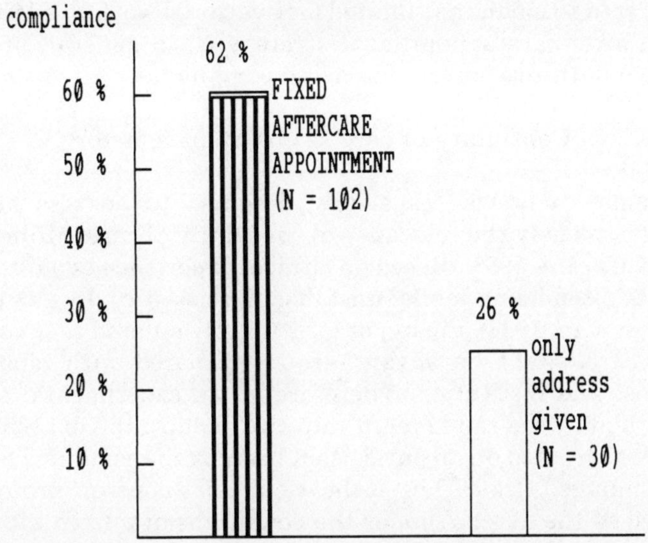

Figure 2: Evaluation of compliance factors (N = 132)

in this study. Compliance was highly correlated ($p < 0.001$) with the arrangement of a fixed after-care appointment (Figure 2), whereas other significant associations, e.g. with socio-demographic characteristics, motivation, diagnostical groups etc., were not demonstrated.

Increased motivational work as compliance factor

In another study (Möller *et al.* 1987; Kurz *et al.* 1988), we tried to answer the question whether additional motivational work could increase compliance under the conditions of a fixed after-care appointment. To keep in close touch with the reality of the usual care situation, the motivational work was intended to be only short: the patients filled out a self-rating questionnaire on motivation (Torhorst *et al.* 1988). On the basis of this information, an additional interview (up to half an hour), performed by the managing psychiatrist, focused on apparent motivational deficits. In addition, the patients received a motivating letter or a phone call from the doctor to ensure that they accepted the after-care recommended. The result was disappointing: only a small but statistically not significant increase to 60 per cent (N = 150) under study conditions as compared with 50 per cent under the situation without special motivational work. This result can be interpreted to mean that limited motivational work in addition to a fixed after-care appointment strategy is, in general, not very effective with respect to increasing compliance.

Continuity of care as compliance factor

The same study was especially designed to address another question, namely the relevance of continuity of care (Möller *et al.* 1987; Kurz *et al.* 1988). Based on clinical experience of parasuicide patients often being labile, unstable, narcissistic, shy etc. (Dietzfelbinger *et al.* 1988), the hypothesis was formulated that continuity of care might be advantageous compared with change of therapist and institution. Therefore, in an experimental design, the patients were randomised into two groups: the experimental group was treated on an out-patient basis by the same psychiatrist who managed their hospitalisation; the control group was referred to the 'Arche' under the conditions of a fixed after-care appointment. The result is quite convincing (Figure 3): 72 per cent

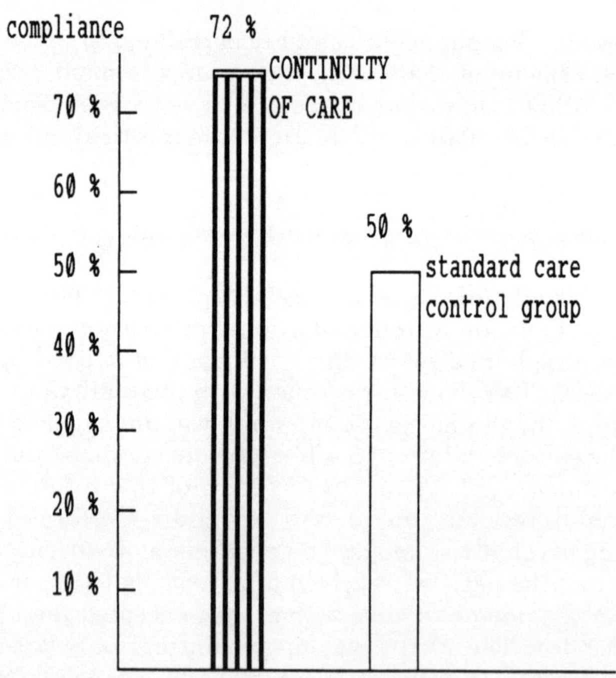

Figure 3: Evaluation of continuity of care (N = 141)

of the experimental group did accept the first session of after-care treatment compared with 50 per cent of the control group ($p < 0.001$). This result demonstrates that even the relatively high compliance under the conditions of a fixed after-care appointment can be greatly surpassed by the addition of greater continuity of care. Furthermore, the data show that the higher degree of compliance in the experimental group was not compensated by higher drop-out rates during after-care treatment. In fact, 38 per cent of the experimental group remained in therapy for more than five sessions, whereas only 12 per cent of the control group did so.

As a side aspect of this study, we found that with this clientele, the physician with the longest psychiatric and psychotherapeutic experience demonstrated the best results regarding compliance.

Time structure of after-care sessions as a compliance factor

In the study under discussion, the twelve sessions of after-care were offered during the three months directly following the parasuicide. Thus, the patients received, in general, one session per week. If necessary, the sessions could be arranged more frequently in the first weeks after parasuicide.

In a recent study (Torhorst *et al.* 1988) devoted to hypothesised special needs of a sample of parasuicide repeaters, we tried to compare in an experimental control group design a similar after-care program, i.e., twelve sessions of short therapy or crisis intervention during three months, with another type of after-care: one session per month over a period of one year. The latter approach was based on the idea that for this special group of parasuicide repeaters, a long-term contact might be preferable to a typical crisis-oriented short psychotherapy. The result demonstrated clearly that compliance was much higher in the crisis-oriented three-month-therapy, whereas there was a considerable drop-out rate in the first month during the long-term contact (Figure 4).

Rating motivation as predictor of compliance

In our second study on compliance we had noted that patient motivation as estimated by a standardised global judgement during hospital stay is not associated with compliance (Möller and Geiger, 1981).

In our large parasuicide study on compliance and motivation

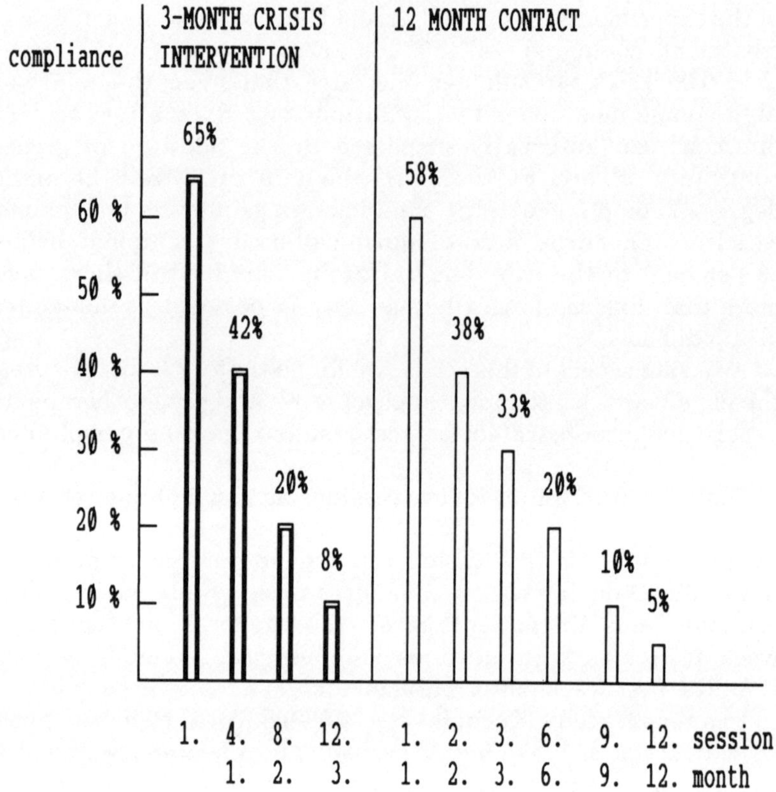

Figure 4: Crisis intervention (N = 40) compared with twelve-month contact (N = 40)

we tried to analyse this aspect more in detail (Möller *et al.* 1987; Torhorst *et al.* 1988). For this study, a global interview rating with seven global categories and a differentiated (fifty-two items) self-rating scale for the standardised assessment of motivation was constructed. These assessment instruments took into account a multidimensional construct of motivation. A principal component analysis of the self-rating scale resulted in the following factors: positive attitude for therapy, subjective obstacles to psychotherapy, previous experience with psychotherapy, no problems from the subjective viewpoint.

Neither the global scores nor the subscores correlated with compliance in this large group of 226 patients. Of the background factors, patients who were more disturbed in terms of depression and anxiety scored higher in motivation. Self-ratings and ratings by the psychiatrist were not closely correlated. Closer correlations (r = 0.20–0.45) were found only between the first self-rating factor and most of the categories of ratings by the doctor.

From these results one would like to conclude that motivation of parasuicide patients assessed at the time of hospital stay seems not to be an important predictor of compliance. Therefore, each patient for whom after-care seems to be indicated should be offered after-care independent of his estimated motivation.

Other background factors for compliance

During our large study on compliance and motivation we also analysed socio-demographic and psychiatric variables with respect to compliance. The following characteristics were correlated with compliance:

- male
- older age (40–59)
- history of psychiatric treatment
- more suicidal thoughts
  (*a*) in the history of the patient
  (*b*) before the index parasuicide
- somewhat more psychopathological disturbances reflected by different scales.

Conclusion

The main results of these empirical studies can be summarised as follows:

(*1*) Compliance of parasuicide patients depends very strongly on different variables of the care system, not only on patients' characteristics.

(*2*) Each patient for whom after-care seems to be indicated should be offered after-care independent of his or her assumed motivation.

(*3*) Especially in problematic cases, compliance with after-care can be increased, among other things, by a fixed after-care appointment, by at least weekly sessions and, if possible, by continuity of care.

References

Bogard, M. (1970). Follow-up Study of Suicidal Patients Seen in Emergency Room Consultation. *American Journal of Psychiatry*, 126 1017–20.

Dietzfelbinger, T., Kurz, A., Torhorst, A. and Möller, H.J. (1988). 'Description and Prognostic Value of Standardized Procedures for Determining Remarkable Personality Traits in Patients Following a Suicide Attempt', in H.J. Möller, A. Schmidtke and R. Welz (eds.), *Current Issues of Suicidology* Berlin: Springer, pp. 328–40.

Graupe, S.R. (1975). 'Ergebnisse und Probleme der quantitativen Erforschung traditioneller Psychotherapieverfahren', in H. Strotzka (ed.), *Grundlagen, Verfahren, Indikationen.* Urban & Schwarzenberg, pp. 32–85.

Häfner, H. (1978). Psychiatrische Krisenintervention—Umsetzung in psychiatrischen Einrichtungen. *Neurologische Psychiatrie (Erlangen),* 4, 397–403.

Hankoff, L.D. (1979). Situational categories. In Hankoff, L.D., Einsidler, B. (eds.), *Suicide—theory and clinical aspects.* PSG Publishing Comp., Littleton/Mass.

Hankoff, L.D., Waltzer, H. (1968). A Suicide-prevention Service in a Psychiatric Receiving Hospital Setting. in H.L.P. Resnik (ed.), *Suicidal Behavior. Diagnosis and Management.* Little, Brown and Comp., Boston.

Kurz, A. and Möller, H.J. (1984). 'Hilfesuchverhalten und Compliance von Suizidgefährdeten', *Psychiatrische Praxis,* 11, 6–13.

Kurz, A., Möller, H.J., Bürk, F., Torhorst, A., Wächtler, C. and Lauter, H. (1988). 'Evaluation of an Outpatient Treatment Program for Suicide Attempters in a General Hospital', in H.J. Möller, A. Schmidtke and R. Welz (eds.), *Current Issues of Suicidology*, Berlin: Springer, pp. 414–18.

Linden, M. (1979). 'Therapeutische Ansätze zur Verbesserung von "compliance"', *Nervenarzt*, 50, 109–14.

Möller, H.J. and Geiger, V. (1981). 'Möglichkeiten zur "Compliance"—Verbesserung bei Parasuizidenten', *Crisis*, 2, 122–9.

Möller, H.J., Bürk, F., Kurz, A., Torhorst, A., Wächtler, C. and Lauter, H. (1987). 'An Empirical Study of Different Aftercare Strategies for Patients who Attempted Suicide: The Effect of Psychotherapy on Compliance and Outcome', in R.J. Daly and E.A. Sand (eds.), *Psychological Treatment of Mental Illness: Research Strategies and Design*, Berlin: Springer, pp. 67–76.

Möller, H.J., Werner, V. and Feuerlein, W. (1978). 'Beschreibung von 150 Patienten mit Selbstmordversuch durch Tabletten—unter besonderer Berücksichtigung des Selbstmordverhaltens und der Inanspruchnahme von Beratungsmöglichkeiten für Suizidgefährdete', *Archiv fuer Psychiatrie und Nervenkrankheiten*, 226, 113–35.

Morgan, H.G., Barton, J., Pottle, S., Pocock, H., Burns-Cox, C.J. (1976). Deliberate Self-harm: a Follow-up Study of 279 Patients. *British Journal of Psychiatry*, 128, 361–8.

Murphy, G.E., Wetzel, R.D., Swallow, C.S. (1969). Who Calls the Suicide Prevention Center? *American Journal of Psychiatry*, 126, 314–24.

Oast, S.P., Zitrin, A. (1975). A Public Health Approach to Suicide Prevention. *American Journal of Public Health*, 65, 144–7.

Paykel, E.S., Hallowell, C., Dressler, D.M., Shapiro, D.L., Weissman, M.M. (1974). Treatment of Suicide Attempters. A Descriptive Study. *Archive General Psychiatry*, 31, 487–91.

Slaikeu, K.A., Tulkin, S.R., Speer, D.C. (1975). Process and Outcome in the Evaluation of Telephone Counseling Referrals. *Journal of Consulting Clinical Psychology*, 43, 700–7.

Sudak, H.S., Sawyer, J.B., Spring, G.K., Coakwell, D.M. (1977). High Referral Success Rates in a Crisis Center. *Hospital Community Psychiatry*, 28, 530–32.

Torhorst, A., Bürk, F., Kurz, A., Wächtler, C. and Möller, H.J. (1988). 'Motivation for Compliance with Outpatient Treatment of Patients Hospitalized after Parasuicide', in H.J. Möller, A. Schmidtke and R. Welz (eds.), *Current Issues of Suicidology*, Berlin: Springer, pp. 458–61.

Outcome of suicide attempters with respect to repetition: A six-month follow-up

A. PHILIPPE, J.Y. GAUTIER and M. VERRON

Suicide attempters constitute a high-risk group for repetition. International surveys (Hawton *et al.* 1982; Morgan *et al.* 1976; Myers, 1982; Retterstol, 1973; Wang *et al.* 1985) show the importance of repetition among suicide attempters, and repeaters represent a large minority of hospitalised suicide attempters, with a frequency of 20–40 per cent; there were 41 per cent in our own survey in 1980 (Davidson and Philippe, 1986). These results emphasised the chronicity of suicide pathology.

Follow-up surveys show that repetition risk is particularly high during the year following the key admission, especially within the first three months. The incidence ranges from 10 per cent to 30 per cent.

This work is the first part of a prospective research on a twelve-months period following a suicide attempt, with regard to repetition rate and existence of psychiatric disorders. The goals of the follow-up study are to evaluate the frequency of repetition and to test the predictive factors of repetition which have been pointed out in our previous study. In the present chapter, situated at mid-term follow-up, only repetition will be regarded.

Material and method

Altogether, 403 people were admitted to the hospital in Lorient (Brittany) between 1 October 1986 and 30 September 1987. Among them, eighty-two repeated once or more during the six months after the key admission. There were 490 admissions during this period

The survey has two phases:

(*a*) At the hospital, suicide attempters are interviewed. Data are collected through a questionnaire based mainly on the original questionnaire used in the 1980 survey. It includes various elements: socio-demographic variables, health status and medical records (out-patient and in-patient psychiatric treatment), method used and circumstances of the suicide attempt, data about relatives' health and diseases, patients' pattern of behaviour after the suicide attempt and their relatives' attitude.

(*b*) Six months later a survey is carried out with the medical services and physicians who have been involved in medical treatment given on discharge from the hospital.

In addition to repetition, which will be the main point dealt with here, we note the type of treatment received since the key admission, and the presence of depressive symptoms and their evolution.

The analyses of the differences between groups are based the chi-square test.

Results

Breakdown by age and sex did not yield significant differences (Table 1). The female to male ratio (60 per cent female) and the importance of young people (58 per cent under thirty-five) are commonly reported.

In all, 85 per cent used drugs, which had been prescribed for them three times out of four; 30 per cent had taken alcohol at the time of the act and the level of coma was equal to or superior to two in 12 per cent of cases; 48 per cent were repeaters; 17 per cent had a severe somatic disease; 37 per cent had previously been admitted to a psychiatric department; and 48 per cent presented with a mental illness.

These results are the same as those reported in similar studies. In our survey of 1980, 67 per cent were women and 67 per cent were under the age of thirty-five. Other results were very similar, except for alcohol use, which was less important.

TABLE 1: Breakdown by age and sex, N = 400

	15–19	*20–4*	*25–9*	*30–4*	*35–9*	*40–9*	*50+*	*Total*
Male	12	27	33	22	27	18	17	156
Female	30	37	35	35	36	40	31	244

Outcome at six months

The repetitions were identified through the following two sources:

(*a*) Information about the patients was obtained from medical services and physicians. At the present time 237 questionnaires have been filled out, representing 59 per cent of the suicide attempters. Fifty-seven have made one or two attempts; six have committed suicide.

(*b*) Hospitalisation records have allowed us to identify eighty-two repeaters.

The rate of repetition at six months is 17 per cent among the subjects who have been followed up. When we consider all the suicide attempters admitted to the hospital during the following period, the rate is 20 per cent.

Significant variables of repetition

To clarify the risk factors for repetition over a short period, two subgroups were constituted:

(*a*) the first-ever patients who did not repeat during the survey; and

(*b*) those who did repeat during the survey.

TABLE 2: Significant variables related to repetition (%)

	First-ever	*Repeaters*	
Educational level			
elementary school	38	58	
high school	58	42	$p < .01$
graduate	4	–	
Professional status			
employees and students	50	23	
precarious job	5	11	
unemployed	20	27	
retired, never worked	19	28	$p < .05$
disabled	6	11	.05
Unconsciousness on admission			
level 0 and 1	93	84	
level 2 and more	7	16	$p < .01$
Alcoholism	20	29	$p < .05$
Psychiatric care			
out-patient	28	63	$p < .01$
in-patient	16	44	$p < .01$
Mental illness	41	57	$p < .01$
Alcoholism in relative	30	45	$p < .01$
Mental illness in relative	18	30	$p < .05$

We excluded those who had previously attempted suicide but who did not repeat during the follow-up period. Compared with the repeaters, they showed no significant differences except for two variables: a higher proportion of relatives with a mental disease; and the existence of bereavement in the repeater group.

Repetition of attempted suicide was significantly related to the variables shown in Table 2.

The risk of repetition in the six-month period seems highly correlated to the existence of a mental illness (this includes psychiatric diagnosis and consultation in a psychiatric unit). The importance of family health status is demonstrated. A low level of education and inactivity (unemployment, disability, etc. . . .) are related to repetition. It may be noted that among those employed those who have a precarious job are also at a high risk. The severity of the attempt, evaluated by a coma level equal or superior to two, is also a risk factor.

Data recorded six months after the initial episodes show significant differences between first-ever attempters and repeaters.

Globally the mean number of depressive symptoms (out of a list of nine) is higher for repeaters (3.7–2.5), and there are significant differences for two individual symptoms, namely suicide ideas and social withdrawal.

We compared the 166 patients who were not followed up with the 237 patients who were: we found differences for only three items. The non-followed-up group contained a lower number of retired and disabled persons (9–18 per cent), they had less mental illness diagnosed (44–51 per cent), and they more often denied their acting out (19–8 per cent). Thus the followed-up subjects presented some special features. Their higher frequency of somatic and mental disease could explain why they were more often in contact with physicians and medical services.

Predictive value of significant variables

Our 1980 survey was cross-sectional. Cluster analysis showed the importance of twelve variables correlated with repetition. They

TABLE 3: Symptoms and risk of repetition (%)

	First-ever	*Repeaters*	
Suicide ideas	19	39	$p < .01$
Social withdrawal	27	55	$p < .01$
Three or more depressive symptoms	45	76	$p < .01$

TABLE 4: Specificity, sensitivity and positive predictive value for three scales (%)

	Specificity	*Sensitivity*	*PPV*
Scale with 12 items	80	41	43
Short scale (7 items)	66	55	38
Buglass and Horton's scale	72	45	38

concerned socio-demographic status, plus educational level or unemployment, method and lethality, health status (admission to hospital and mental illness), and characteristics of family environment. A first scale was built up with these twelve variables (cut-off point at four).

Using seven out of the nine most significant variables we also constructed a second scale (cut-off point at three), and we compared these two scales to Buglass and Horton's scale (cut-off point at two) (Buglass & Harton, 1974).

These results concern the 237 patients who were followed up. For specificity, sensitivity and predictive power these three scales produced similar results comparable to those already published, in particular, a level of predictivity lower than 50 per cent.

Discussion

At the present time the data from this survey are only partially analysed. The first results are very similar to those of our previous study and those reported in the international literature. We especially note the importance of psychopathology among suicide attempters who repeat and among their relatives. Socio-demographic variables such as professional status or educational level are significant.

About 60 per cent of all the suicide attempters are seen by medical teams or by physicians within six months of their key admission. Among those who are not seen, most probably prefer to forget their suicide attempt. They have few different characteristics from others. The results of the study by Sakinowsky *et al.* (1979) support this point of view; the authors find a similar attitude among suicide attempters who dropped out from a follow-up survey.

The incidence of repetition is particularly high—20 percent within six months—and is higher than the incidence shown in comparable surveys. Wilkinson and Smeeton (1987) report 16 per cent incidence of repetition for a one-year period. Bancroft and Marsack (1977), during a period of three years, find 26 per cent incidence of repetition, most of them during the first six months. Many studies find less than 10 per cent incidence of repetition in six months. The results of the present analysis cannot totally explain the high repetition rate. Nevertheless, it must be noted that this area of France is one of the regions where suicide incidence is at the highest (70 per cent higher than the national mean incidence), where the incidence of attempting suicide is higher than in our previous survey (25 per cent higher), and where repeaters constitute a larger group (48–41 per cent).

Although repetition is not uncommon, risk scales failed to identify clearly a group of repeaters with a high level of confidence. As reported by Myers (1982) in a critical review of the literature, we too found a relative low level of predictivity.

Conclusion

The prevalence of repetition among suicide attempters admitted to a general hospital is high. A six-month follow-up demonstrates the importance of repetition, and identifies the associated risk factors such as a low socio-cultural level, and health problems (alcoholism and mental illnesses) among the probands and their relatives.

However, an evaluation of the different risk scales shows that they have a low positive predictive value for repetition. This emphasises the difficulty of predicting repetition in individual cases.

References

Bancroft, J. and Marsack, P. (1977). 'The Repetitiveness of Self-Poisoning and Self-Injury', *British Journal of Psychiatry*, 131, 393–400.

Buglass, D., Harton, J. (1974). 'A scale for predicting subsequent suicidal behaviour' *British Journal of Psychiatry*, 124, 573–8.

Davidson, F. and Philippe, A. (1986). 'Suicide et tentative de suicide aujourd'hui. Etude épidémiologique'. Doin/INSERM, Paris, 173 p.

Hawton, K., Fagg, J., Marsack, P. *et al.* (1982). 'Deliberate Self-Poisoning and Self-Injury in the Oxford Area, 1972–1980', *Social Psychiatry*, 17, 175–9.

Morgan, H.G., Barton, J., Pottle, S. *et al.* (1976). 'Deliberate Self-Harm: A Follow-up of 279 Patients', *British Journal of Psychiatry*, 128, 361–8.

Myers, E.D. (1982). 'Subsequent Deliberate Self-Harm in Patients Referred to a Psychiatrist: A Prospective Study', *British Journal of Psychiatry*, 140, 132–7.

Retterstol, N. (1973). 'Personal Follow-up Examination of Patients Admitted to a Psychiatric Hospital', in N. Speyer, R.F.W. Diekstra, K.J.M. van de Loo (eds.), *Seventh International Congress on Suicide Prevention*, Amsterdam, pp. 110–13.

Sakinowsky, J., Streiner, D.L. and Ligate, L. (1979). 'Suicide Attempters One Year Later: The Impact of Changing Life Situations and Systems of Care', in *Proceedings Communications: 10th International Congress for Suicide Prevention and Crisis Intervention, Ottawa*, AIPS, Ottawa, pp. 99–108.

Wang, A.G., Nielsen, B., Bille-Brahe, U. *et al.* (1985). 'Attempted Suicide in Denmark. III: Assessment of Repeated Suicidal Behaviour', *Acta Psychiatrical Scandinavica*, 72, 389–94.

Wilkinson, F. and Smeeton, N. (1987). 'The Repetition of Parasuicide in Edinburgh, 1980–1981', *Social Psychiatry*, 22, 14–19.

Controlled studies of psychosocial intervention following attempted suicide

K. HAWTON

In spite of the recent decrease in deliberate self-poisoning and self-injury in the United Kingdom (Brewer and Farmer, 1985; Platt *et al.*, 1988), rates of this behaviour are still very high, and self-poisoning remains the most common reason for acute medical admission of women to general hospitals and the second most common reason for such admissions of men (Hawton and Catalan, 1987). The importance of careful assessment of suicide attempters in the general hospital is unquestionable. However, there is little consensus about what might be the best policies for after-care of patients who do not require psychiatric hospital admission. For example, the proportions of patients offered out-patient care vary considerably between different clinical services (e.g. Platt *et al.*, 1988). Furthermore, there is no general agreement about which treatment approaches for such patients are most appropriate.

The reasons for this situation are, in part, the dearth of controlled studies of treatment of these patients and, as will be shown, the somewhat disappointing results of the few studies which have been conducted. This chapter presents a review of the prospective randomised controlled treatment studies of attempted suicide patients which have been carried out in the United Kingdom. Only studies of primarily psychosocial intervention are included, not studies solely of the use of medication. In addition to drawing conclusions from the findings of these studies, the problems inherent in such investigations will also be examined. Finally, suggestions will be made about how future treatment studies of attempted suicide patients might be conducted.

Four studies meeting the criteria noted above have been carried out and reported in the literature. The first of these was conducted in Edinburgh, the second in Southampton, and the third and fourth in Oxford. They have not included identical groups of patients and the methods and settings of treatment have varied. These differences have reflected the differing objectives of the separate investigations. However, the four studies are sufficiently comparable to allow general conclusions to be made.

Evaluation of an experimental after-care service for repeaters

This study, conducted in Edinburgh (Chowdhury *et al.*, 1973), was of patients who met the criteria for being called 'repeaters', having a history of at least one parasuicidal act (attempted suicide) before the act which resulted in their inclusion in the investigation. However, for ethical reasons, patients considered to be at especially high risk of a further attempt on the basis of their scores on a predictive scale (Buglass and McCulloch, 1970) were excluded from the comparative study.

Following their assessment in hospital, patients suitable for the study were randomly assigned to either an experimental after-care service or to a control treatment.

Experimental after-care service

Patients assigned to the experimental after-care service group were offered regular and frequent out-patient appointments; those who did not keep an out-patient appointment were visited at home without delay. An emergency telephone call service was available, and home visits were also made in response to emergency calls. The service was staffed by a full-time psychiatrist and a social worker, with assistance from two part-time social workers.

Control treatment

Patients assigned to this treatment group were offered routine follow-up from the hospital psychiatric service, but none of the special facilities of the experimental after-care programme. Typically, patients in this group were offered an out-patient appointment to see a psychiatrist and/or social worker, but non-attenders were not pursued.

Results

The design and results of this study are summarised in Table 1. As can be seen, there was no difference between the two treatment groups in the proportion of patients who made further attempts

TABLE 1: Evaluation of an experimental after-care service for repeaters*

	Number of patients	*% repeating attempts during 6-month follow-up*
	No.	%
Experimental after-care service	71	24
Regular and frequent out-patient appointments		
Domiciliary visits		
24-hour emergency call service		
Control treatment	84	23
Out-patient appointments (non-attenders not pursued)		

* Chowdhury *et al.*, (1973).
Social circumstances (finance, housing, employment) improved in more of those in the experimental after-care service group with social problems at the outset than in those in the control group (63% compared with 31%), but this effect was largely confined to women (76% compared with 36%), with men benefiting relatively little extra from the experimental after-care service (42% compared with 26%).

during the six months after entering the study. However, social circumstances were improved in more of those in the experimental group than in the control group, but this apparent effect of the experimental after-care service was largely confined to women.

Evaluation of a social work after-care service for self-poisoning patients

In this study, conducted in Southampton (Gibbons *et al.*, 1978), an experimental social work after-care service was compared with routine after-care. Self-poisoning patients referred to a general hospital were initially assessed by a psychiatrist and then included in the study unless they were suffering from a formal psychiatric illness requiring immediate psychiatric treatment, or were judged on the basis of a scale to be an immediate suicide risk, or were in continuing treatment with a psychiatrist or social worker whom they had seen recently. The suitable patients were allocated randomly to either the experimental social work after-care service or to the control treatment group.

Experimental social work after-care service

Patients in this group were offered help in their own homes by one of two social workers who used the treatment approach called task-centred casework (Reid and Epstein, 1972), in which the therapist tries to help the patient to tackle specific tasks relevant to their key problem. This treatment lasted for up to three months. The social worker was available at times of crisis.

Control treatment: routine care

Patients in the control treatment group were offered routine care (i.e. referral back to their general practitioners, psychiatric referral, or other referral).

Results

The nature of the two treatment groups and the results of the study are summarised in Table 2. There was no difference between the rates of repetition of self-poisoning in the two treatment groups during the year following entry to the study. Although depression scores (measured on the Beck Depression Inventory: Beck *et al.*, 1961) had improved considerably for patients in both treatment groups by the time of the four-months follow-up, there was no difference in the degree of change in scores between the

TABLE 2: Evaluation of a social work atter-care service for self-poisoning patients*

	Number of patients	*% repeating attempts within one year of entry to study*	*Depression after 4 months*	*Social problems after 4 months*
	No.	%		
Social work after-care service				
Up to 3 months social work intervention at home	200	13.5		86% of patients improved
Task-centred casework for specific problems				
Social worker available at times of crisis			No difference	$p < 0.02$
Traditional care				
Referral back to GP (54%) or				70% of patients improved**
Psychiatric referral (33%) or Other referral (13%)	200	14.5		

* Gibbons *et al.* (1978).

** The beneficial effects of the social worker service on social problems were confined to women (Gibbons, 1979).

two groups. However, social problems were more often reported as improved by patients in the social work intervention group. When the two sexes were examined separately, this apparent beneficial effect of social work intervention on social problems was confined to women (Gibbons, 1979). It should be noted that the ratings of social problems were based on how the patients viewed their overall social circumstances. This raises the possibility that there may have been an attributional effect rather than a real treatment effect in the social work intervention group, although this would have to have applied only to the female patients. By the time of an 18-months follow-up no differences in outcome were found between the two treatment groups on any of the measures (Gibbons, 1979).

Domiciliary compared with out-patient treatment of self-poisoning patients

Because of the rather poor compliance found with out-patient care, especially the relatively high non-attendance rate, a home-based treatment programme was developed in Oxford for some self-poisoning patients. Subsequently, a treatment study was conducted to compare the relative efficacy of home-based (domiciliary) and out-patient treatment (Hawton *et al.*, 1981). The actual style of treatment, which was brief (one to ten sessions) problem-orientated counselling (Hawton and Catalan, 1987), was the same in the two treatment conditions, except that appointments in the domiciliary regime could be offered on a flexible time schedule whereas those for patients in the out-patient group were confined to a weekly out-patient clinic.

Patients included in the study were those who, after a careful initial assessment in hospital following their overdoses, were judged suitable for out-patient care. Assignment to treatment groups was on a randomised basis. Treatment for patients in both groups was provided by either of two psychiatrists, a social workers, or a psychiatric nurse, all of whom had considerable previous experience of treating such patients.

Results

A summary of the design of the study and the results is provided in Table 3. In spite of far better compliance in the domiciliary treatment group, with almost twice as many patients in this group

TABLE 3: Domiciliary versus out-patient treatment of self-poisoning patients*

	Domiciliary treatment		*Out-patient treatment*
	Home-based *Problem-orientated counselling* *Flexible schedule of appointments*		*Out-patient appointments* *Problem-orientated counselling* *Weekly out-patient clinic*
Number of patients	48		48
Treatment completed	83%	($p < 0.001$)	42%
Repetition of attempts within 1 year of entry to study	10%	(NS)	15%
Mood (post-treatment, and 6-months follow-up)		No difference between groups	
Social adjustment (post-treatment and 6-months follow-up)		No difference between groups	
Target problems (post-treatment and 6-months follow-up)		No difference between groups	

* Hawton *et al.* (1981).

completing treatment, and extensive overall improvement in ratings of patients' mood, social adjustment, and target problems during the follow-up period, there were no major differences in outcome between the two groups. Patients with problems in their relationship with a partner at entry to the study were significantly more improved in the domiciliary treatment group at the six-month follow-up in terms of their marital relationship ratings on the Social Adjustment Scale (Weissman and Paykel, 1974, modified as per Hawton, 1979). The outcome data have recently been re-analysed for the two sexes separately. Unlike in the two previous studies, no differential effect between the two treatments was found for the two sexes, in spite of the fact that female patients more often attended treatment sessions than did male patients.

No difference in outcome was found between patients treated by the two psychiatrists and those treated by the two non-medical therapists. This finding added weight to the growing opinion that assessment and after-care of self-poisoning patients could be adequately provided by well-trained and supervised non-medical staff, a policy which subsequently was incorporated in new Department of Health and Social Security Guidelines for the management of these patients (DHSS, 1984).

The negative findings of this study with regard to the effectiveness of domiciliary compared with out-patient treatment resulted in the home treatment programme of the Oxford service largely being abandoned because of the considerable extra expense and time involved in seeing people in their own homes. However, the out-patient programme was developed further to include flexible timing of out-patient appointments rather than a weekly schedule, and continuity of care for the individual patient with control being maintained with the same professional throughout assessment and after-care; these factors appear to improve compliance with out-patient care (Hawton *et al.*, 1979).

Out-patient counselling compared with general practitioner care for self-poisoning patients

Following the failure to find any major difference in efficacy between home-based and out-patient treatment of self-poisoning patients, the natural next step was to evaluate out-patient counselling itself, compared with a less intensive treatment. Therefore, a further study was mounted in Oxford, in which out-patient care was compared with returning patients to the care of their general practitioners (Hawton *et al.*, 1987). Following a thorough assessment in the general hospital, self-poisoning patients judged suitable for out-patient counselling were randomly assigned to the two treatment conditions.

Out-patient counselling

Patients in this condition received problem-orientated counselling (Hawton and Catalan, 1987), including conjoint treatment with a partner where this seemed appropriate. All treatment sessions took place in out-patients, appointments being arranged on a flexible basis. Treatment was brief (one to eight sessions), and was provided by one of five experienced non-medical counsellors (four psychiatric nurses, one social worker).

General practitioner care

Patients assigned to this group were returned to the care of their general practitioners with advice being provided to the doctors on possible help they might provide or arrange.

Results

The content of treatment and the results are summarised in Table 4. As in the previous three studies, no major differences in repetition rates was found between the patients in the two treatment groups. Similarly, there was no difference in outcome with regard to depression scores (Beck Depression Inventory). There were, however, some non-significant trends on social adjustment scores and outcome of target problems suggesting rather better outcome for the out-patient group, although the differences were non-significant. Overall, therefore, there was little evidence to suggest that out-patient counselling was markedly superior to general practitioner care.

However, some interesting and predicted findings emerged when subgroups of patients were examined. First, women seemed to benefit more from out-patient counselling than general practitioner care, especially in terms of the outcome of their target problems. At the 4-month assessment there were several other trends in support of this statistically significant finding. Rates of compliance with out-patient care had been rather better among female than male patients. Secondly, patients with dyadic problems (i.e. problems in a relationship with a current partner)

TABLE 4: Out-patient counselling versus general practitioner care for self-poisoning patients*

	Out-patient counselling		*General practitioner care*
	Brief, problem-orientated counselling *Conjoint treatment if appropriate* *Flexible out-patient appointments* *Non-medical therapists*		*Discharge to care of general practitioner with treatment recommendations*
Number of patients	40		40
Repetition of attempts during 1 year after entry to study	7%	(ns)	15%
Depression (2, 4, and 9 months after entry to study)		No difference between groups	
Social adjustment (2, 4, and 9 months after entry to study)		(ns, but trends favouring (out-patient group)	
Target problems 2, 4, and 9 months after entry to study)		(ns, but trends favouring (out-patient group)	

* Hawton *et al.* (1987).
Women and patients with *dyadic problems* benefited more from outpatient care.

had somewhat better outcome if they were part of the out-patient counselling group. The differences in outcome between these patients and those in the general practitioner group were marked at the 9-months follow-up, especially with regard to depression scores, target problems, and overall social adjustment scores.

Summary of the findings from the controlled treatment studies

Several conclusions can be drawn from the findings of the four treatment studies of attempted suicide patients which have been considered.

(*1*) There is no evidence that any type of psychosocial intervention evaluated so far has a preventive effect against repetition of attempts.

(*2*) Although home-based treatment increases attendance at treatment sessions, it does not significantly increase the overall effectiveness of treatment.

(*3*) In three out of four studies special treatment programmes appeared to have beneficial effects for women, especially in terms of their social adjustment. There is no evidence that special after-care programmes have extra benefits for men.

(*4*) In the two studies in which they were specifically examined, patients with dyadic problems appeared to gain benefit from special after-care programmes, although this was not marked until six to nine months after entry to treatment.

Problems and difficulties in treatment studies of attempted suicide patients

When the treatment studies of attempted suicide patients are reviewed, it is clear that there are considerable problems and difficulties in implementing a truly satisfactory study. Thus, there are difficulties concerning the nature of the patient population, how treatment is delivered, how a comparative study is established and maintained, and the methods of assessment of outcome. These are considered in more detail below on the basis both of the studies that have already been described and of others in the literature.

Characteristics of subjects included in investigations

By their nature, attempted suicide patients constitute a very heterogeneous population, having in common a single behaviour (a suicide attempt), not a specific psychiatric disorder. The range of problems experienced by these patients is vast, including difficulties due, for example, to relationship problems, family problems, loss, unemployment, personality problems, alcohol abuse and so on (Hawton and Catalan, 1987, pp. 26–36). Such wide variation means that:

(*1*) specific type of treatment is unlikely to be appropriate, let alone effective, for all patients;

(*2*) there is bound to be very large statistical variance in scores on assessment measures (e.g. mood and social adjustment scales) such that the chances of detecting positive effects of treatment are very limited.

Evaluation of intervention against a background of crisis resolution

For most patients, considerable improvement occurs in their mood and social adjustment soon after their attempts, even if no treatment is provided. This reflects the fact that crisis situations tend to resolve, at least to some degree, this often being the direct result of the attempt itself (Hawton and Catalan, 1987, pp. 46–8). Because treatment studies have to be conducted against this background of rapid change, the chances of detecting treatment effects, which may be relatively small, are again limited. The situation is very different for studies of treatment of conditions which are more persistent (e.g. agoraphobia, obsessional disorders).

Size of treatment groups

As a consequence of the first two problems, the size of treatment groups may have to be unmanageably large (several hundred subjects) if treatment effects are going to be detected in studies of very heterogeneous populations of attempters.

Definition and limits of treatment approaches

In some treatment studies, the actual treatment approaches have been inadequately described, so that it has been difficult or impossible for other workers, both clinical and research, to try them out themselves. This obviously limits the value of such studies. It has also often proved difficult to define boundaries to treatment approaches which are being compared, so that there is no, or little, overlap between them. If there is too much overlap, then treatment effects may again be obscured.

Maintenance of separation between treatment groups

Even if there is clear demarcation between treatment groups at the outset, it may be difficult to maintain this separation as a study proceeds. For example, if one group of patients is allocated to a 'no treatment' group (usually this is unacceptable because it is unethical) or 'minimal treatment' condition, it may be impossible to restrict the patients to this condition because, for example, some patients will seek out help themselves (e.g. from general practitioners, voluntary or other agencies) or a further attempt may result in help being offered.

Inappropriate outcome measures

The outcome measures used in some studies have been of questionable validity. For example, results obtained with a global self-report measure of social adjustment might reflect the attention received by the patients from their therapists rather than indicate true treatment effects.

Compliance with research assessments

Some attempted suicide patients prove difficult to follow up, partly because of the inherent high mobility of this population and partly because of negative attitudes to being followed up, especially over a long period.

Suggestions for future treatment studies

Further treatment studies of attempted suicide patients are clearly required. However, the problems and difficulties discussed above must be addressed if such studies are going to help in the search for more effective means of helping these patients. The following are some suggestions as to how future treatment studies can be designed in order to overcome some of the problems that have been highlighted.

Subjects

It is likely that the most useful information about effective treatment approaches will be obtained from studies which focus on specific target populations of patients, not simply all attempters. Appropriate groups might be very high-rate repeaters (i.e. one or more previous attempts), those who are at risk of repetition, women, and patients with dyadic problems. New treatment approaches for male attempters need to be developed and evaluated.

It is also important that future investigations include sufficient numbers of subjects to allow treatment effects to be detected. Power estimation based both on known characteristics of the group being studied and typical change scores in outcome measures following attempts should be carried out before a study is launched in order to gauge the numbers of subjects necessary to detect meaningful clinical differences. Where very large numbers are indicated, a multi-centre study might be considered, but such an investigation is usually difficult to mount satisfactorily.

Intervention

The content of treatment being offered must be appropriate to the target population. Problem-solving (Hawton and Catalan, 1987, pp. 88–132; Hawton and Kirk, 1989) appears to be an approach most suited to many attempted suicide patients. Conjoint therapy, using similar principles, is likely to be effective for patients with dyadic problems. Whatever treatment approach is chosen, this must be fully described so that other workers can apply it in their work.

Assessment of outcome

The measures used to assess outcome must be carefully chosen, and outcome assessments should be carried out at time intervals likely to allow detection of treatment effects.

In choosing assessment measures, attention should be paid to their relevance both to the target population and treatment approaches being studied. A battery of measures, including (in addition to repetition of attempts) assessment of changes in target problems (see Hawton *et al.* 1981, 1987), mood (e.g. Beck Depression Inventory: Beck *et al.* 1961), social adjustment (e.g. Social Adjustment Scale: Cooper *et al.*, 1982), suicidal ideas (e.g. Suicide Ideation Scale: Beck *et al.*, 1979), and attitudes to treatment, will usually be satisfactory.

Taking into account the rapid changes which often occur in the period immediately following an attempt, the high risk of repetition during this early phase (Bancroft and Marsack, 1977), and the likelihood that treatment will be relatively brief, it is important that the first outcome assessment is timed to detect any immediate treatment effects. An initial assessment one to three months after the attempt is, therefore, appropriate. Subsequent assessments might be conducted at four to six months, and then at nine to twelve months after the attempts. In some patients, especially those with dyadic problems, there is reason to expect that treatment effects may not become apparent until the later assessments.

Conclusions

The results of controlled studies of treatment of attempted suicide patients have so far been somewhat disappointing. No experimental treatment based on psychosocial intervention has been shown to affect the rate of repetition of attempts. However, there is some evidence of benefit in terms of social adjustment, although this effect appears to be confined to women and, possibly, to patients with dyadic problems. Further work is needed to identify methods of helping male attempters.

Treatment research with this population of patients is bedevilled by several problems and difficulties. Future studies of treatment for these patients is clearly required. However, if such studies are to be productive, it is imperative that the lessons which can be learnt from previous investigations are taken into account when planning further research in this area.

References

Bancroft, J. and Marsack, P. (1977). 'The Repetitiveness of Self-Poisoning and Self-Injury', *British Journal of Psychiatry*, 131, 394–9.

Beck, A.T., Ward, C.H., Mendelson, M., Monk, J. and Erbaugh, J. (1961). 'An Inventory for Measuring Depression', *Archives of General Psychiatry*, 4, 53–63.

Beck, A.T., Kovacs, M. and Weissman, A. (1979). 'Assessment of Suicidal Intention: The Scale for Suicidal Ideation', *Journal of Consulting and Clinical Psychology*, 47, 343–52.

Brewer, C. and Farmer, R. (1985). 'Self-Poisoning in 1984: A Prediction that didn't Come True', *British Medical Journal*, 290, 391.

Buglass, D. and McCulloch, J.W. (1970). 'Further Suicidal Behaviour: The Development and Validation of Predictive Scales', *British Journal of Psychiatry*, 116, 483–91.

Chowdhury, N., Hicks, R.C. and Kreitman, N. (1973). 'Evaluation of an Aftercare Service for Parasuicide (Attempted Suicide) Patients', *Social Psychiatry*, 8, 67–81.

Cooper, P., Osborn, M., Gath, D. and Feggetter, G. (1982). 'Evaluation of a Modified Self-Report Measure of Social Adjustment', *British Journal of Psychiatry*, 141, 68–78.

DHSS (1984). *The Management of Deliberate Self-Harm.* HN (84), 25, London: Department of Health and Social Security.

Gibbons, J.L. (1979). *The Southampton Parasuicide Project*, Report to the DHSS, Department of Psychiatry, Royal South Hants Hospital, Southampton.

Gibbons, J.S., Butler, P., Urwin, P. and Gibbons, J.L. (1978). 'Evaluation of a Social Work Service for Self-Poisoning Patients', *British Journal of Psychiatry*, 133, 111–18.

Hawton, K. (1979). 'Evaluation of Short-Term Psychiatric Intervention, following Acts of Self-Poisoning', DM thesis: University of Oxford.

——Bancroft, J., Catalan, J., Kingston, B., Stedeford, A. and Welch, N. (1981). 'Domiciliary and Out-Patient Treatment of Self-Poisoning Patients by Medical and Non-Medical Staff', *Psychological Medicine*, 11, 169–77.

Hawton, K. and Catalan, J. (1987). *Attempted Suicide: A Practical Guide to its Nature and Management*, 2nd ed., Oxford: Oxford University Press.

Hawton, K., Gath, D.M. and Smith, E.B.O. (1979). 'Management of Attempted Suicide in Oxford', *British Medical Journal*, 141, 166–70.

Hawton, K. and Kirk, J. (1989). 'Problem-Solving', in K. Hawton, P. Salkovskis, J. Kirk and D.M. Clark (eds.), *Cognitive Behaviour Therapy for Psychiatric Problems: A Practical Guide*, Oxford: Oxford University Press.

Hawton, K., McKeown, S., Day, A., Martin, P., O'Connor, M. and Yule, J. (1987). 'Evaluation of Outpatient Counselling Compared with General Practitioner Care Following Overdoses', *Psychological Medicine*, 17, 751–61.

Platt, S., Hawton, K., Kreitman, N., Fagg, J. and Foster, J. (1988). 'Trends in Parasuicide in Edinburgh and Oxford, 1976–1984', *Psychological Medicine*, 18, 405–18.

Reid, W. and Epstein, L. (1972). *Task-centered Casework*, New York: Columbia University Press.

Weissman, M.M. and Paykel, E.S. (1974). *The Depressed Woman: A Study of Social Relationships*, Chicago: University of Chicago Press.

Factors affecting therapeutic decision-making following a suicide attempt

R. ZUMBRUNNEN and L. TRICOT

Introduction

Assessment and therapeutic orientation of suicidal patients accounts for an important part—both quantitatively and qualitatively—of the activity of most psychiatric consultation–liaison units in general hospitals. The significance and seriousness of self-harmful acts are quite different from one patient to another, therefore clinical assessment and decision depend on many variables. Numerous suicidology articles and textbooks provide guidelines for clinical assessment and management of suicidal patients (Hawton and Catalan, 1987, pp. 58–87; Kreitman, 1986, pp. 181–95; Gunn-Sechehaye, 1986, pp. 77–91). Other authors propose standardised rating scales as an aid to clinical evaluation and prediction of suicidal behaviour (Resnick, 1980, Patterson *et al.*, 1983; Victoroff, 1983, pp. 67–77; Motto *et al.*, 1985; Poeldinger, 1983). Another interesting approach, which is beginning to arouse interest among clinicians and researchers, consists of studying the determinants of psychiatric decision-making (Hermann, 1984).

The present study was conducted in order to investigate the impact of some factors on therapeutic decision-making following a suicide attempt. A recent research overview (Marson *et al.* 1988) stressed the multiplicity of variables related to clinical decision in the emergency room: influences (and interactional influences) such as demographic, clinical and those of clinician, family and health system were reviewed. Unfortunately, emergency room psychiatric pathology is very heterogeneous, and no study specifically devoted to the decision-making process following suicidal behaviour could be found in the literature.

In the Canton and City of Geneva (area population 360 000),

most persons making a suicide attempt (requiring in-patient care) are admitted to the emergency room of the University General Hospital. They are referred to the consultant psychiatrist as soon as the somatic emergency is cleared.

The emergency room is staffed with three part-time psychiatric registrars, from the consultation–liaison unit, who are trainees in their third or fourth years. They are there for a six- or twelve-month rotation, and are supervised by a senior psychiatric fellow. There is no specially trained psychiatric nurse, and the formal administrative responsibility remains with the physician. Night and week-end wards are alternately assumed by one of the ten registrars of the consultation–liaison unit. The clinical assessment is careful and thorough as far as is permitted by the emergency room rule (twenty-four hours maximum stay), and is summarised in a semi-standardised consultation report. The spectrum of possible choices is as follows (from the least to the most restrictive):

(*a*) *discharge home with no actively planned follow-up*, which includes conditions where no therapeutic indication exists, and conditions where there is a relative indication, but no patient motivation;

(*b*) *actively organised out-patient follow-up*, including possibility of treatment by the consultant him or herself;

(*c*) *admission (voluntary) to the Brief Therapy Centre (BTC)*, intermediate psychiatric structure, half-crisis centre, half-day centre, situated in the city, outside the general hospital;

(*d*) *admission (voluntary or involuntary)* to the psychiatric hospital, situated 10 km from the general hospital;

(*e*) *admission to the medical or surgical ward of the general hospital*—a special case, since this decision is generally imposed by the seriousness of the physical injury and is not the psychiatrist's choice.

Patients, material

All patients aged 16–65 years admitted after a suicide attempt and psychiatrically examined during the calendar year 1986 were included. 'Suicide attempt' was defined according to Schneider's definition, as 'a missed suicide, whatever the reason for the failure could be: inappropriate method, intervention of a third person, successful treatment, etc.'. This concept of suicide attempt includes the (usually) conscious intent of self-killing, with 'death as a means or as an end' (Schneider, 1954).

For each consultation regarding suicide attempt, the following variables from the consultation report were recorded:

socio-demographic variables: sex, age, nationality

anamnestic variables: suicidal method, presence/absence of significant others at admission time

health system variables: kind of pre-admission treatment (if any), patient's place of residence (as the three public psychiatric sectors have a precisely defined catchment area and their own care policy)

diagnostic variable: psychiatric diagnosis according to DSM III

decision variable: therapeutic orientation after assessment—no follow-up/out-patient therapy/admission to BTC/admission to psychiatric hospital/admission to general hospital for more than one week.

Method

The following data were analysed:

– contingency tables concerning the first (during 1986) suicide attempt of each considered patient;

– individual data for the twenty-two patients who made at least two suicide attempts during the year of observation.

The contingency tables were the object of correspondence analysis, then of tests of independence. The individual data permitted control of the stability of the conclusions over time.

Correspondence analysis

This method (Benzecri, 1973; Caillez and Pages, 1976) is a descriptive statistical instrument which allows the display of existing correspondences between many variables. Significant correspondences appear graphically obvious. Numerical results led to the selection of variables ('socio-demographic', 'clinical', and 'health system') possibly related to 'decision'. Associations were eventually tested through statistical tests.

Tests of independence

We examined contingency tables in which one of the margins is fixed, corresponding to the variable where the influence on the decision was tested. Chi-square tests were used on tables with more than two rows or more than two columns, concerning the first suicide attempt. We referred to exact tests of independence in 2×2 tables, using an asymptotically normal statistic: t (Kendall and Stuart, 1973, pp. 573–4).

Taking into account multiple suicide attempts

If a patient makes multiple attempts during the period of observation, certain variables concerning the patient may change:

suicidal method;
pre-admission treatment;
presence of significant others at admission;
psychiatric diagnosis;
therapeutic orientation (decision);
and place of residence.

These changes led to modifications in the contingency tables constructed on the basis of the first suicide attempt. Each modified 2 × 2 table considering multiple attempts could be tested, and the conclusion could change from one table to another. Significance was given to results which were stable over time.

Results

Epidemiological data

During the year 1986, 402 interventions for suicide attempt, relating to 374 patients, were performed and included in the study. The general characteristics of the material are given in Table 1. The female to male ratio was 2:1, and the mean age of the patients was thirty-three (s.d. 11) years. Suicide attempt 'repeaters' were similarly distributed according to sex and age.

Calculation of the suicide attempt rate in Geneva had to take into account additional data: forty-three suicide attempt patients

TABLE 1: General characteristics of material

	Patients (N = 374)		*Attempts (N = 402)*	
	N	%	N	%
Number of attempts				
1	352	94	352	87
> 1	22	6	50	13
Sex				
male	121	32	131	33
female	253	68	271	67
Age				
15–24	107	29	111	28
25–44	195	52	214	53
45–65	72	19	77	19

were examined by the pedopsychiatric and psychogeriatric consultants; approximately 10 per cent of admitted suicide attempters were not psychiatrically examined (premature discharge), and around 10 per cent were admitted to another (private) hospital. Thus, the suicide attempt rate for the Geneva population in 1986 can be estimated at 490 for 360 000, i.e., 134 per 100 000 per year, while the completed suicide rate was 25 per 100 000 in the same year (Fryc, 1987).

Global data concerning therapeutic decision

Table 2 shows the breakdown of therapeutic decisions on discharge from the emergency room. Out-patient after-care was the most frequent decision taken, followed by 'no follow-up', in other words no actively organised treatment. The recently created Brief Therapy Centre was used in 15 per cent of cases, just a little less than the psychiatric hospital. Only 5 per cent of patients had to be hospitalised for more than one week in the general hospital. Comparisons with published results from other European countries are difficult because of differences in mental health systems (Hawton and Catalan, 1987; Platt *et al.* 1988; Meran-Conrie *et al.* 1987). Nevertheless, the rate of psychiatric admission seems higher in Geneva than that in Britain, but comparable to that of France.

Association between 'socio-demographic factors' and 'decision'

Table 3 shows that the association between 'age' and 'decision' was statistically significant ($p < 0.001$) regarding the first suicide attempt. Under twenty-five years, patients were preferably oriented to out-patient therapy (exact test: $t = 3.27$, $p < 0.001$, no change over time); those aged 25–44 years were often sent to the BTC ($t = 3.19$, $p < 0.001$); while older patients (45–65) were fre-

TABLE 2: Breakdown of therapeutic decisions

	Patients (N = 374)		*Attempts (N = 402)*	
	N	%	*N*	%
No follow-up	109	29	113	28
Out-patient therapy	121	32	129	32
Brief therapy centre	54	15	56	14
Psychiatric hospital	70	19	80	20
General hospital	20	5	24	6

TABLE 3: Association between 'age' and 'decision'

Age	*No follow-up (N = 109)*	*Out-patient (N = 121)*	*BTC (N = 54)*	*Psychiatric hospital (N = 70)*	*General hospital (N = 20)*
	N	*N*	*N*	*N*	*N*
15–24	36	48	6	13	4
25–34	35	24	23	17	6
35–44	19	31	16	21	3
45–65	19	18	9	19	7

chi-square = 33.548; df = 12; $p < 0.001$

quently admitted to the psychiatric or the general hospitals ($t = 2.66$, $p < 0.05$).

Male patients were more often hospitalised, while women were more often admitted to the Brief Therapy Centre, but there was overall association between 'sex' and 'decision' (chi-square = 6.283 df = 4). 'Nationality' (Swiss as against 'foreigner' patients) and 'decision' were also unrelated.

Association between 'anamnestic factors' and 'decision'

Figure 1 displays the correspondences between 'decision' and the 'anamnestic' and 'health system' variables.

The figure is divided into three zones depending on the therapeutic orientation:

(*a*) above left: the general hospital, close to the most 'violent' methods of suicide used,

(*b*) to the right: absence of orientation (no follow-up) close to absence of pre-admission treatment (none) and attempted suicide by benzodiazepine ingestion (benzo intox),

(*c*) below left: all the instances of psychiatric treatment, follow-up and decision taken, close to other drug abuse (other intox) and phlebotomy.

There was a global dependence between the 'suicidal method' and the subsequent decision: benzodiazepine ingestions often left the hospital with no follow-up, concerning women ($t = 4.61$, $p < 0.001$), while other drug intoxications seem to have been considered more serious by the consultants, as they actively organised out-patient therapy for these patients. Violent suicidal methods (mechanical, chemical, physical) frequently led to follow-up especially for women ($t = 2.04$, $p < 0.05$) and led to hospitalisation for both sexes ($t = 8.33$, $p < 0.001$). The global association between 'method' and 'decision' is confirmed by the chi-square test (Table 4). These results moderate the previously stated absence of influence of 'sex' and 'decision'.

TABLE 4: Association between 'suicidal method' and 'decision'

Method	*No follow-up (N = 109)*	*Out-patient (N = 121)*	*BTC (N = 54)*	*Psychiatric hospital (N = 70)*
	N	*N*	*N*	*N*
BDZ intox	48	37	25	15
Other intox	44	62	20	37
Other method	17	22	9	18

chi-square = 14.44; df = 6; $p < 0.05$

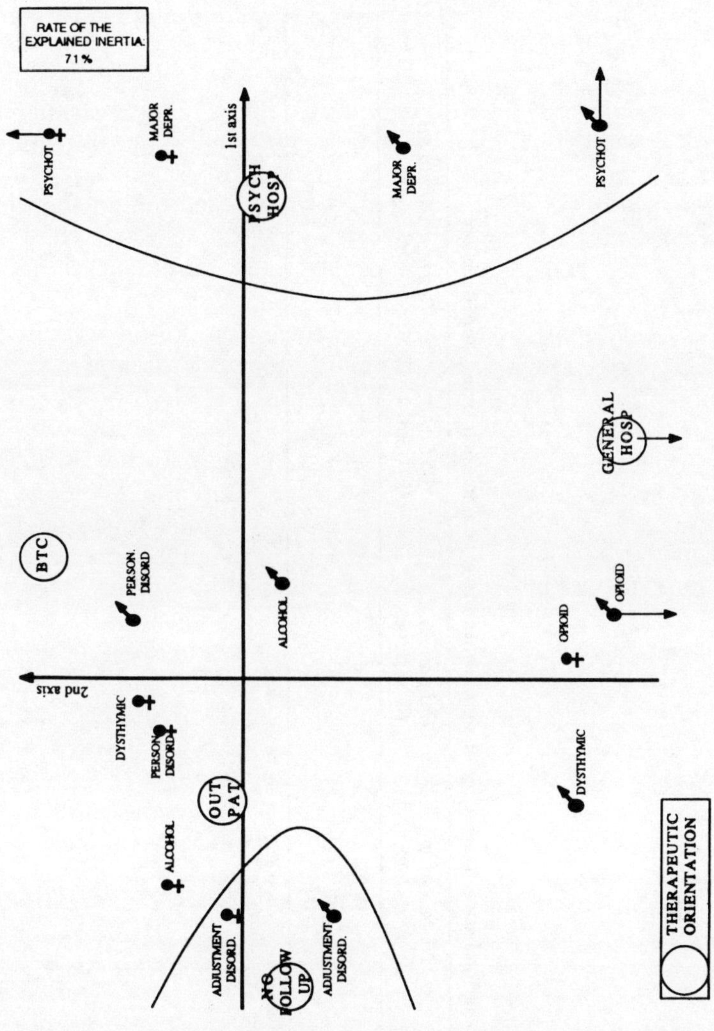

Figure 1: 'Decision': 'anamnestic', and health system

TABLE 5: Association between 'presence of significant others' at admission time,* and 'decision'

Significant others	*No follow-up (N = 100)*	*Out-patient (N = 110)*	*BTC (N = 50)*	*Psychiatric hospital (N = 64)*	*General hospital (N = 15)*
	N	*N*	*N*	*N*	*N*
Present	70	76	38	33	4
Absent	30	34	12	31	11

* For this variable, information was available for only 339 patients
chi-square = 19.42; df = 4; $p < 0.001$

Another anamnestic factor was significantly associated with 'decision': 'presence of significant others' at admission time (Figure 1 and Table 5). Patients with no 'significant other' were more often hospitalised, but were infrequently sent to the Brief Therapy Centre.

In Table 5, no follow-up was organised for 100 patients, of whom seventy were accompanied at admission by significant others. Of these, fifty-three were female and seventeen were male patients; in this subgroup of patients, the female to male ratio was significantly higher than in the total sample.

'Health system' factors and 'decision'

There was a global dependence between 'decision' and 'kind of pre-admission treatment' (or, more precisely, 'kind of therapist'). The association (Figure 1) is statistically significant (Table 6). The majority (66 per cent) of patients who were not under treatment at the time of the attempt left the hospital with no follow-up planned. Patients of physicians were often sent to the BTC, and patients of private and public psychiatrists were frequently admitted to the psychiatric hospital. Despite differences in psychiatric care policies among the three psychiatric sectors, especially regarding admission criteria in the Brief Therapy Centres, there was no significant association between 'place of residence' (determining attribution to one sector) and 'decision' (chi-square = 10.018 df = 8).

'Diagnostic factors' and 'decision'

Figure 2 and Table 7 summarise the results. A significant association was found between 'decision' and three DSM III diagnoses or diagnostic categories: patients with major depression or psychotic disorders (essentially schizophrenic disorder) were, for the most part, admitted to the psychiatric hospital; patients with adjustment disorders very often left the hospital with no-follow-up. Other frequent diagnostic categories were alcohol abuse/dependence, opioid abuse/dependence, dysthmic disorder, and Axis II personality disorders. Decision distribution for the patients in these diagnostic categories did not differ significantly from the global distribution.

It is to be noted that female patients always figure in a higher part of the diagram than male patients, except for the personality disorders diagnosis. This result underlines the fact that women

TABLE 6: Association between 'kind of pre-admission treatment' and 'decision'

Pre-admission Treatment	*No follow-up (N = 109)*	*Out-patient (N = 121)*	*BTC (N = 54)*	*Psychiatric hospital (N = 70)*	*General hospital (N = 20)*
	N	*N*	*N*	*N*	*N*
None	62	16	4	9	3
Physician	34	35	26	13	10
Private psychiatrist	9	33	9	20	3
Public psychiatrist	4	37	15	28	4

chi-square = 116.65; df = 12, $p < 0.001$

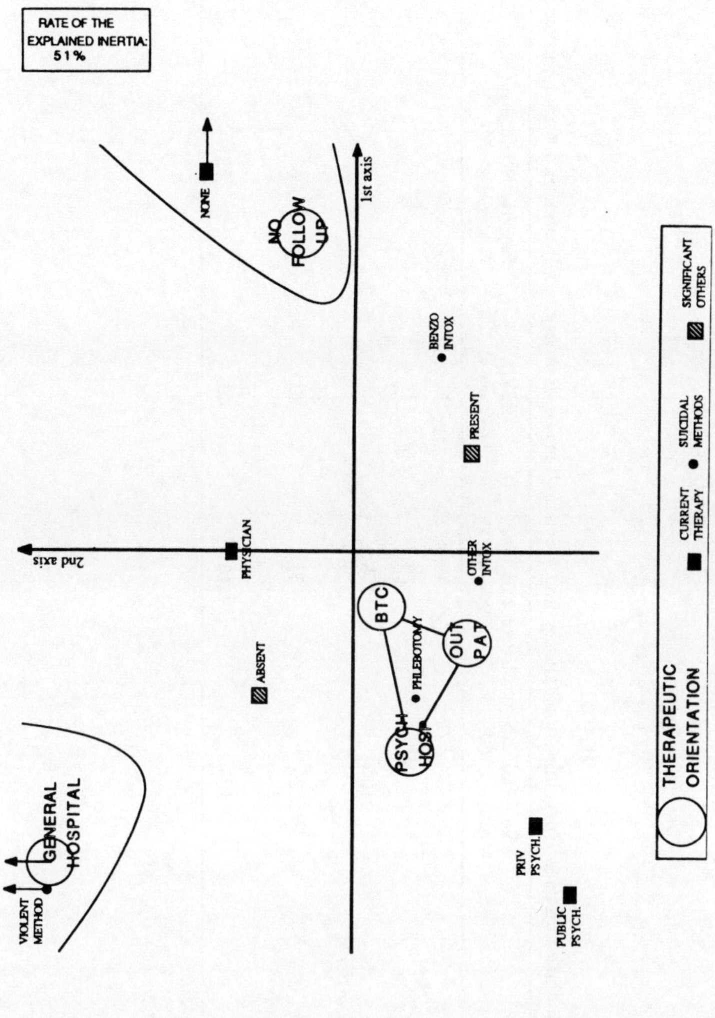

Figure 2: 'Decision':, diagnostic factors

TABLE 7: Association between 'psychiatric diagnosis' and 'decision': major depression, adjustment disorders, psychotic disorders

	No follow-up (N = 109)	*Out-patient (N = 121)*	*BTC (N = 54)*	*Psychiatric hospital (N = 70)*	*General hospital (N = 20)*
	N	*N*	*N*	*N*	*N*
*Major depression**					
yes	5	16	20	30	7
no	104	105	34	40	13
*Adjustment disorder***					
yes	81	67	25	17	9
no	28	54	29	53	11
*Psychotic disorder****					
yes	1	5	5	12	2
no	108	116	49	58	18

* Chi-square = 53.183; df = 4, $p < 0.001$
** Chi-square = 44.843; df = 4, $p < 0.001$
*** Chi-square = 20.271; df = 4, $p < 0.001$

are more often oriented to BTC, and men to general hospital. This observation is true whatever the Axis I psychiatric diagnosis.

Discussion

Epidemiological data were drawn from the study due to the fact that the Geneva General Hospital receives the vast majority of all suicide attempts committed in the Geneva area. The estimated suicide attempt rate (134 per 100 000 per year), as well as sex and age distribution, are comparable with results from other European countries, despite different recording methods and definitions (Diekstra, 1982, pp. 1–16; Vedrinne *et al.* 1981, pp. 114–27; Plat *et al.* 1988). Nevertheless, the need for internationally recognised criteria and definitions of suicidal behaviour is urgent. In our unit, where DSM III is used as the routine diagnostic system, 'suicide attempt' was introduced as an additional code on DSM III Axis I, with subcategories according to the type of suicidal method and to the intensity and degree of certitude of suicidal intent.

Regarding decision-making and the influence of various factors on therapeutic orientation, our study tried to combine the statistical inference (tests) with a descriptive multivariate approach (correspondence analysis). Several variables proved to be significantly associated with the subsequent therapeutic decision. Among 'socio-demographic' variables, 'age' was a major determinant: the older the patients, the more the decision was restrictive and institutional. This finding is consistent with the notion of a higher risk of completed suicide among older persons than among young people. There was no global dependence between 'sex' and 'decision', apart from the observation that the general hospital received a small group mostly composed of men, and that the newly created Brief Therapy Centre received a large majority of female patients. This finding will lead us to discuss with our colleagues in charge of the BTCs the possible factors preventing the admission of male patients.

Among the 'health system' variables, the type of care-givers previously chosen by the patient was strongly associated with the subsequent 'decision'. Above all, the impressive finding was that 66 per cent of the patients undergoing no treatment at the time of the suicide attempt were leaving the hospital with no-follow-up planned. These untreated and possibly unwilling patients deserve further study. Longitudinal surveys could prove to be useful to evaluate the spontaneous prognosis of these patients, and the eventual need for new therapeutic strategies especially designed for them. Distribution of decisions appeared quite similar for patients treated by psychiatrists, either from the private or public sector. Interestingly, the decision profile for the physicians' patients seems to be situated somewhere between the profile for the psychiatrists' patients and the profile for the untreated patients. This result offers attractive perspectives for research on the characteristics of each mental health provider's patients.

Finally, certain 'psychiatric diagnoses' are highly associated with therapeutic orientation. As expected, major depression and psychotic disorders are correlated with psychiatric hospitalisation. More surprisingly, adjustment disorders are significantly associated with no follow-up. These reactive pathologies are less severe than major psychiatric disturbances. Nevertheless, the patients suffer from manifest crisis states. Perhaps the psychiatrists are not yet prepared and trained to provide the simple and often punctual counselling intervention this kind of patient needs. Other frequent diagnoses (personality disorders, dysthmic disorder, alcohol and opioid abuse and dependence) were characterised by profiles of decision similar to each other and to the entire sample. This result indirectly suggests (or confirms the clinical impression) that these pathologies share a common denominator with each other and with the suicide attempt behaviour.

References

Benzecri, J.P. (1973). *L'analyse des données*, vol. 2, Paris: Dunod.

Caillez, F. and Pages, J.P. (1976). *Introduction à l'analyse des données*, Paris: SMASH.

Diekstra, R.F.W. (1982). *Suicide in EEC*, Basel: Karger, Biblthca Psychiatry, 162.

Fryc, O. (1987). Personal communication, Medico-Legal Institute, University of Geneva.

Gunn-Sechehaye, A. (1986). 'Eléments de suicidologie', in *Manuel de Psychologie Médicale Propédeutique*, Geneva: Médicine et Hygiène.

Hawton, K. and Catalan, J. (1987). 'Assessment of Patients after Deliberate Self-Poisoning or Self-Injury', in *Attempted Suicide: A Practical Guide to its Nature and Treatment*, Oxford: Oxford Medical Publications.

Hermann, P. (1984). 'La prise de décision médicale', *Psychologie Médicale*, 16, 599–604.

Kendall, M.G. and Stuart, A. (1973). *The Advanced Theory of Statistics*, 3rd edn., vol. 2, London: Griffin.

Kreitman, N. (1986). 'The Clinical Assessment and Management of the Suicidal Patient', in A. Roy (ed.), *Suicide*, Baltimore: Williams and Wilkins.

Marson, D.C., McGovern, M.P. and Pomp, H.C. (1988). 'Psychiatric Decision Making in the Emergency Room: A Research Overview', *American Journal of Psychiatry*, 145, 918–25.

Meran-Conrie, N., Leger, J.M., Malauzat, D. *et al.* (1987). 'Etudes épidémiologiques des conduites suicidaires', *Psychologie Médicale*, 19, 685–7.

Motto, J., Heilbron, D. and Juster, R. (1985). 'Development of a Clinical Instrument to Estimate Suicide Risk', *American Journal of Psychiatry*, 142, 680–6.

Patterson, W.M., Dohn, H.H., Bird, J. and Patterson, G.A. (1983). 'Evaluation of Suicidal Patients: The Sad Persons Scale', *Psychosomatics*, 24, 343–9.

Platt, S., Hawton, K., Kreitman, N., Fagg, J. and Foster, H. (1988). 'Recent Clinical and Epidemiological Trends in Parasuicide in Edinburgh and Oxford: a Tale of Two Cities', *Psychological Medicine*, 18, 405–18.

Poeldinger, W. (1983). 'Dix erreurs possibles dans le traitement des patients suicidaires et dépressifs', *Bulletin Médicins Suisses*, 64, 691–4.

Resnick, H.L.P. (1980). 'Psychiatric Emergencies' in H. Kaplan, A. Freedman and B. Sadock (eds.), *Comprehensive Textbook of Psychiatry* 3rd edn., vol. 2, Baltimore: Williams and Wilkins.

Schneider, P.B. (1954). *La tentative de suicide*, Neuchâtel: Delachaux et Niestlé.

Vedrinne, O., Quenard, D. and Weber, D. (1981). *Suicides et conduites suicidaires: Aspects socioculturels, épidémiologiques*, vol. 1, Paris: Masson.

Victoroff, V. (1983). *The Suicidal Patient: Recognition, Intervention, Management*, New-Jersey: Oradell.

Acknowledgement

We thank Dr C. Aubry for her assistance with the English translation.

6

SPECIAL STUDIES

The early impact of bereavement after suicide or fatal traffic accident

J. VAN DER WAL, M.P.H.D. CLEIREN, R.F.W. DIEKSTRA and B.J.M. MORITZ

In recent years there has been a growing interest in bereavement after suicide (see, for example, Dunne *et al.*, 1987). At least three reasons can be suggested for this attention. First, suicide is a cause of death that attracts attention since it is an extremely complex phenomenon. Menninger (1959) has drawn attention to this by pointing out that in suicide the elements of dying, killing, and murder are represented. Not surprisingly, suicide leads to violent and diverse reactions, such as horror and condemnation, but also respect and sympathy. Secondly, in the last few decades rates of suicide have been rising dramatically, leaving a correspondingly increasing number of relatives and friends to mourn. Thirdly, there is a strong suggestion in the literature that suicidal loss is an especially severe form of bereavement. It is said that the grief process is relatively more complicated and of longer duration (Shneidman, 1972; Schuyler, 1973; Praeger and Bernhardt, 1985). More specifically, the standard image of bereavement after suicide contains, among others, the following assumptions (Van der Wal, 1987):

(*a*) strong feelings of guilt;
(*b*) social stigmatisation and loss of social support;
(*c*) a never-ending search for explanations; and
(*d*) an increased chance of suicidal behaviour among survivors.

This standard image, or 'suicide survivor syndrome' as it is sometimes called (McIntosh, 1987), can be disputed, however. It is based largely on clinical observation, anecdotal information, and theoretical speculation. However, there is no sound empirical evidence for the assumption that a suicidal death is more devastating for survivors than other causes of death.

TABLE 1: Unique characteristics of bereavement by suicide

(*a*)	A search for motives which the deceased may have had for committing suicide
(*b*)	Intra-psychic denial of the cause of death
(*c*)	Feeling rejected by the deceased
(*d*)	Religious questions regarding the fate of the deceased after taking his own life
(*e*)	Concealment of the cause of death in contacts with others
(*f*)	Fear of being susceptible through heredity to the same psychological problems as the deceased

A recent review of the literature (Van der Wal, 1987) revealed that bereavement after suicide is qualitatively different from bereavement after other causes of death in several respects (Table 1). It must be pointed out that these characteristics do not generally occur. Moreover, the question remains to what extent the specific characteristics of suicidal loss influence the grief process and the quality of adjustment to the loss.

In this study, attention will be paid to some of the aspects of psychological and social adaptation to bereavement after suicide compared with bereavement after another form of unnatural death, namely a fatal traffic accident.

Method

Subjects

The sample consisted of ninety-one survivors of people who committed suicide and ninety-three survivors of people who died after a fatal traffic accident. They were all close relatives of the deceased. Some characteristics of the study groups are listed in Table 2.

TABLE 2: Characteristics of subjects

	Survivors of suicides (N = 91)					*Survivors of traffic fatalities (N = 93)*				
	Sex			*Age*		*Sex*			*Age*	
Kinship	*M*	*F*	*Total*	*Mean*	*s.d.*	*M*	*F*	*Total*	*Mean*	*s.d.*
Parent	7	11	18	57	(12.3)	14	14	28	52	(10.5)
Spouse	5	9	14	43	(18.4)	6	12	18	44	(18.6)
Sibling	19	16	35	39	(16.1)	13	15	28	32	(17.3)
Child	15	9	24	41	(9.3)	6	13	19	30	(5.9)
Total	46	45	91	44	(16.4)	39	54	93	40	(15.2)

Suicides were documented in co-operation with participating police forces who gave us access to their files. Fatal traffic accidents were documented in co-operation with local health authorities and from newspaper reports. In this way an un-selected sample was formed of all suicidal deaths and traffic fatalities which occurred in the research area.

Two months after the loss, relatives of all deaths were invited by letter and phone to participate in the study. Only those survivors aged eighteen years and over were invited. The response rate for each study group was 66 per cent. Survivors were interviewed on average about four months after their loss (M = 112 days, s.d. = 23.5 days).

Instruments

The study instrument covered a broad range of demographic, relational, and loss characteristics and of psychological, social, and practical consequences of the loss. Only a few of the social and psychological consequences of the loss will be discussed here.

Indices of *psychological adjustment* were as follows:

the short version of the Beck Depression Inventory (BDI-13, Beck and Beck, 1972), used to estimate the degree of depression;

the Leiden Bereavement Scale (LBS), to measure a crucial aspect of recovery from bereavement, that is difficulty with detachment from the deceased;

the Relief Scale (RS) to give an indication of the occurrence of feelings of relief after the loss;

the Guilt Scale (GS), to measure feelings of guilt; and

search for meaning (SfM) was investigated with one question. All instruments were specially developed for this study, with the exception of the BDI.

The indices of *social well-being* were also developed for this study. Results of three of them will be discussed:

the Emotional Support Scale (ESS), to measure the need for (NESS), as well as the satisfaction with, emotional support (SESS);

the Experienced Social Avoidance Scale (ESAS), to give an indication of the extent to which signs of ignorance and avoidance are experienced in social contacts.

An evaluation of both content-related validity and criterion-related validity of these instruments yielded satisfactory results.

Results

Socio-demographic characteristics

The socio-demographic characteristics of both study groups were remarkably similar, with some exceptions for age of survivors (sisters, sons, and daughters of persons who died after suicide being older than their counterparts in the group of survivors of traffic fatalities), and age of deceased (those who died after suicide were younger than the traffic fatalities in the survivor groups of fathers and sisters). However, after analysis of covariance, these differences proved to be not meaningful.

Anticipation of the loss

For 43 per cent of the survivors of suicides the loss was unexpected, 35 per cent expected it to some degree, and for 12 per cent the suicide was not at all unexpected. For survivors of traffic fatalities the loss was always completely unexpected.

Health and psychological problems of those who died

Both groups differed markedly in the health and psychological problems of those who died, as reported by the survivors (Table 3). Almost all survivors of suicides reported more or less serious mental problems among those who died. Among those who died in a traffic accident, only a minority had such problems. The same trend, although not so strong, can be observed with regard to health problems.

Psychological and social adjustment

Both survivor groups were compared according to the already-mentioned indices of psychological and social adjustment by means of multivariate analysis of variance. Exploration of the data had made clear that kinship and sex were closely related to psychological and social well-being of survivors. Therefore, it was decided to include both variables as factors in the MANOVA, next to the cause of death. The essential findings are listed in Table 4.

TABLE 3: Psychological and health problems of those who died, as reported by survivors of suicides and traffic fatalities

	Psychological problems		*Health problems*	
	S	*TF*	*S*	*TF*
	%	%	%	%
None	9	71	37	73
Mild	9	20	10	14
Moderate	10	7	7	7
Severe	72	2	45	7

Note:
S = suicides
TF = traffic fatalities

TABLE 4: MANOVA for the effects of cause of death, kinship, and sex on indices of psychological and social adjustment

	Source of Variation (F values)						
	Cause of death (A)	*Kinship (B)*	*Sex (C)*	$A \times B$	$A \times C$	$B \times C$	$A \times B \times C$
Multiv. effect	15.43***	2.59***	1.67	1.47	0.58	1.27	1.27
Univar. effect							
LBS	11.39***	10.47***	6.77**	2.73*	0.37	3.85*	2.75*
BDI	0.03	5.85***	7.93**	2.51	1.33	1.68	0.15
GS	51.42***	7.38***	0.14	2.00	1.38	0.86	0.76
RS	44.78***	0.90	0.03	0.60	0.34	1.30	0.54
SfM	0.22	4.23**	2.22	1.48	0.89	0.73	1.43
NESS	0.40	1.99	5.22*	0.84	0.55	5.60**	2.00
SESS	0.08	0.87	0.98	0.63	0.19	1.39	1.53
ESAS	0.06	4.59**	0.00	1.09	0.39	1.85	1.41

***$p < 0.001$
**$p < 0.01$
*$p < 0.05$

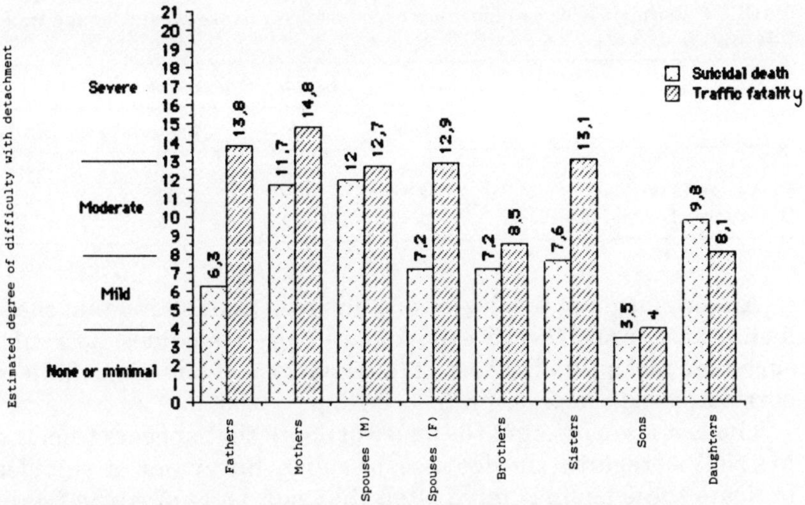

Figure 1: Mean scores on the Leiden Bereavement Scale, by cause of death, kinship, and sex

The main and interaction effects of cause of death, kinship, and sex will be discussed in turn.

When we look at the effects of the *cause of death* firstly, significant differences are found for difficulty with detachment from the deceased, feelings of guilt and relief. Further analyses resulted in the following findings.

Survivors of traffic fatalities show more difficulty with detachment from the deceased than the other survivor group. These differences are especially clear within the groups of fathers and sisters of deceased (Figure 1). The cause of death has also a main effect on the Guilt Scale, survivors of suicides exhibiting greater guilt (Table 5).

TABLE 5: An estimation of the degree of feelings of guilt for survivors of suicides and traffic fatalities, by kinship

		Estimated degree of feelings of guilt			
		None	*Mild*	*Moderate*	*Severe*
		%	%	%	%
Parents	(S)	17	33	50	–
	(TF)	75	14	7	4
Partners	(S)	36	50	14	–
	(TF)	83	17	–	–
Siblings	(S)	37	49	12	3
	(TF)	79	21	–	–
Children	(S)	54	42	4	–
	(TF)	95	5	–	–

TABLE 6: Estimated degree of feelings of relief for survivors of suicides and traffic fatalities

	Estimated degree of relief			
	None	*Mild*	*Moderate*	*Strong*
	%	%	%	%
Survivors of suicides	41	17	20	23
Survivors of traffic fatalities	85	7	6	3

An estimation of the degree of feelings of guilt shows that these feelings are rarely severe, even for survivors of suicides. As a rule, survivors feel guilty because of (alleged) acts of omission. Guilt is correlated with depression ($r = 0.28$, $p < 0.001$).

The last main effect of the cause of death that appears from the MANOVA regards the feelings of relief. Survivors of suicides indicate these feelings more often than survivors of traffic fatalities (Table 6). The reason for relief is most often that the suicidal person is no longer suffering. Relief is negatively correlated to difficulty with detachment ($r = -0.28$, $p < 0.001$).

It is interesting to note that feelings of guilt and relief are not correlated ($r = 0.09$, n.s.). This is contrary to the often-mentioned suggestion that relief is a source of feelings of guilt (Rudestam and Agnelli, 1987).

The factor *kinship to the deceased* appears to be most important in understanding grief reactions. Parents and partners have the highest scores on the LBS (difficulty with detachment from the deceased), the BDI (depression; Table 7), the GS (guilt; Table 5) and are most occupied with the search for meaning (Table 8). Adult children show the least intense grief reactions, while

TABLE 7: Estimated degree of depression for kinship and sex, according to norms as established by Beck and Beck (1972)

	Estimated degree of depression			
	None or minimal	*Mild*	*Moderate*	*Severe*
	%	%	%	%
Fathers	67	14	14	5
Mothers	36	20	32	12
Partners (M)	36	46	9	9
Partners (F)	57	14	19	5
Brothers	91	6	3	–
Sisters	52	23	16	10
Sons	86	10	5	–
Daughters	68	14	14	4

TABLE 8: The degree to which survivors are occupied with the search for meaning, by kinship

	Being occupied with the search for meaning	
	Not/Sometimes	*Often/Continually*
	%	%
Parents	43	57
Partners	59	41
Siblings	78	22
Children	81	19

siblings are roughly midway between. There is also an effect of kinship on the Experienced Social Avoidance Scale. Here partners indicate problematic social interactions most often, followed by parents, siblings, and children (Figure 2). These scores may also be interpreted as an indication of the vulnerability of survivors to unpleasant social interaction, such as being avoided.

The negative social reactions which are discussed here were mentioned by 81 per cent of the partners, 74 per cent of the parents, 73 per cent of the siblings, and 53 per cent of the children. The frequency with which they do occur is, however, not very high. It is also noteworthy that these reactions usually come from people with whom they do not have very close contacts. This is probably the reason why survivors as a rule felt not very offended by them.

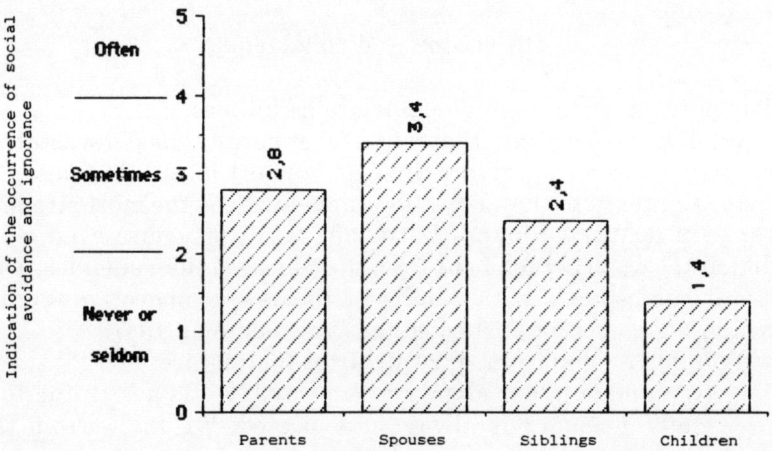

Figure 2: Mean scores on the Experienced Social Avoidance Scale, by kinship

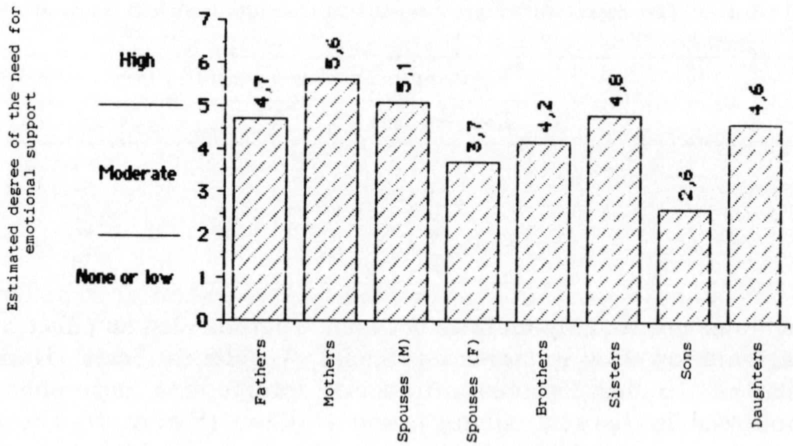

Figure 3: Mean scores on the Need for Emotional Support Scale, by kinship and sex

Finally, *gender* appears to be related to several indices of adjustment. Women have more difficulty with detachment from the loss (Figure 1). This effect is most clear within the groups of siblings and children. Women report also higher depression scores (Table 7) and a higher need for emotional support, but an exception must be made for partners, where men have a higher need for emotional support than women (Figure 3). No effects were found on the Satisfaction with Emotional Support Scale. As a rule, survivors were reasonably satisfied with the emotional support they had received.

Discussion and conclusions

The most important conclusions are as follows.

(*a*) The assumption that suicide generally has devastating consequences for survivors finds no support in our findings.

(*b*) Contrary to the suggestion that suicide is the most stressful cause of death, we found that traffic fatalities cause even more difficulties with detachment from the deceased than suicides. This result corresponds with results of the few comparative studies which have been published so far (Van der Wal, 1987).

Possible explanations for the latter finding are:

(i) suicide is not always unexpected, while a loss due to a traffic accident is always unexpected. We know from the literature that, as a rule, unexpected loss causes more violent grief-reactions (Ball, 1977; Parkes and Weiss, 1983).

(ii) The relation between survivors and those who died is more often troubled in the case of suicide than is the case of traffic fatalities. We can assume from the relevant literature that such difficulties weaken the closeness of ties (Spanier and Lewis, 1980). Consequently, detachment from the loss may be less difficult. This hypothesis remains to be tested, however.

(iii) Many survivors of suicide react with relief because the suicidal person is no longer suffering. Contrary to what is often assumed, this is no cause of feelings of guilt, and it makes detachment from the loss sometimes less difficult.

(*c*) Survivors of suicide more often report feelings of guilt. Even though we found a meaningful correlation with depression, survivors of suicide are not more depressed than survivors of traffic fatalities. One explanation for this finding is that feelings of guilt are usually not very intense. Another possible explanation is offered by the literature on causal attributions. Van den Bout (1986) found that it is not the direction of attributions (that is to say, attributing the cause to one's self versus to others) that is important for adjustment to a loss, but the degree to which one is occupied with attributional activity. So it is possible that survivors of traffic fatalities are more engaged in attributing the cause to others than survivors of suicides, but that this also is related to depression. This hypothesis also remains to be tested.

(*d*) It appears that suicide does not lead to a relatively more complicated process of social adjustment. The groups did not differ with regard to the need for, and satisfaction with, emotional support, and experiences with ignorance and social avoidance.

(*e*) In understanding reactions to the loss, the factor kinship is more important than the cause of death. Generally speaking, parents have most difficulty with the psychological adjustment, followed closely by partners. Grown-up children show the least intense grief reactions, while siblings take up a middle position. With regard to social adjustment, this picture is roughly the same, with the exception that partners have more difficulty in coping with social adaptation than have parents.

These findings also correspond to results of studies in which the bereavement of several kinship groups has been compared (Owen *et al.* 1982–3; Sanders, 1979–80; Lehman *et al.* 1987).

Our conclusions refer to short-term effects of the loss. The question can be raised, of the significance of our findings for long-term adjustment. In this respect, it is important to note that the short-term reaction to a loss is a reliable predictor for adjustment in the future (Parkes and Weiss, 1983; Zisook and Devaul, 1983; Johnson *et al.* 1986).

In the foregoing discussion, the severity of suicide as a risk factor in bereavement has been put in perspective, by means of a comparison with loss after traffic fatalities. This in no way is meant to minimise the severity of bereavement after suicide. Rather, it stresses the fact that bereavement as such is a risk factor in the development of social, psychological, and physical problems (Stroebe and Stroebe, 1987). However, these risks must not be exaggerated in the case of suicidal loss so that all survivors of suicide have to expect devastating consequences. This can lead survivors to worry unnecessarily, and care-givers can react with over-anxiousness. In both cases, the much-feared 'suicide survivor syndrome' can become a self-fulfilling prophecy.

References

Ball, J.F. (1977). 'Widows' Grief: The Impact of Age and Mode of Death', *Omega*, 7, 307–33.

Beck, A.T. and Beck, R.W. (1972). 'Screening Depressed Patients in Family Practice', *Postgraduate Medicine*, December, 81–5.

Bout, J. van den (1986). *Verliesgebeurtenissen in àttributie theoretisch perspectief*, Delft: Eburon (with abstract in English).

Dunne, E.J., McIntosh, J.L. and Dunne-Maxim, K. (eds.) (1987). *Suicide and its Aftermath: Understanding and Counseling the Survivors*, New York and London: Norton.

Johnson, R.J., Lund, D.A. and Dimond, M.F. (1986). 'Stress, Self-Esteem and Coping During Bereavement among the Elderly', *Social Psychology Quarterly*, 49, 273–9.

Lehman, D.R., Wortman, C.B. and Williams, A.F. (1987). 'Long-term Effects of Losing a Spouse or Child in a Motor Vehicle Crash', *Journal of Personality and Social Psychology*, 52, 218–31.

McIntosh, J.L. (1987), 'Research, Therapy and Educational Needs', in E.J. Dunne, J.L. McIntosh and K. Dunne-Maxim (eds.), *Suicide and its Aftermath: Understanding and Counseling the Survivors*, New York and London: Norton.

Menninger, K. (1959). 'Psychoanalytic Aspects of Suicide'. in *A Psychiatrists World: Selected Papers of Karl Menninger*, New York: Viking.

Owen, G., Fulton, R. and Markusen, E. (1982–3). 'Death at a Distance: A Study of Family Survivors', *Omega*, 13, 191–225.

Parkes, C.M. and Weiss, R.S. (1983). *Recovery from Bereavement*, New York: Basic Books.

Praeger, S.G. and Bernhardt, G.R. (1985). 'Survivors of Suicide: A Community in Need', *Family and Community Health, The Journal of Health Promotion and Maintainance*, 8, 62–72.

Rudestam, K.E. and Agnelli, P. (1987). 'The Effect of the Content of Suicide Notes on Grief Reactions', *Journal of Clinical Psychology*, 43, 211–18.

Sanders, C.M. (1979–80). 'A Comparison of Adult Bereavement in the

Death of a Spouse, Child and Parents', *Omega*, 10, 303–21.
Schuyler, D. (1973). 'Counselling Suicide Survivors: Issues and Answers', *Omega*, 4, 313–21.
Shneidman, E.S. (1972). 'Foreword' in A.C. Cain, (ed.), *Survivors of Suicide*, Springfield, Ill: Charles C. Thomas.
Spanier, G.B. and Lewis, R.A. (1980). 'Marital Quality: A Review of the Seventies', *Journal of Marriage and the Family*, November, 825–39.
Stroebe, W. and Stroebe, M.S. (1987). *Bereavement and Health: The Psychological and Physical Consequences of Partner Loss*, Cambridge: Cambridge University Press.
Wal, J. van der (1987). 'The Aftermath of Suicide: A Review of Empirical Evidence', paper presented at the 1 Congresso Nazionale sullo Studio e la prevenzione del Suicidio, Padova, Italy.
Zisook, S. and DeVaul, R.A. (1983). 'Grief, Unresolved Grief and Depression', *Psychosomatics*, 24, 247–56.

Suicides in West Berlin (1981–1985): Reliability of Data

N. HEIM

Introduction

The initial aim of this study on completed suicides in West Berlin was to check or replicate research findings published mainly in American literature about suicides of physicians, who are supposed to have a higher suicide rate than the average population or other related professions (Steppacher and Mausner, 1974; Rose and Rosow, 1982). The fact that professional or occupational variables are not included in official statistics made it necessary to use another data reference system, i.e., access to police or prosecution files was needed. Among other variables, these documents include professional or occupational data for coding, whatever the validity and reliability of these data may be. The results reported here are based on differences that were found between official statistics and the prosecutional suicide data collected.

Methods and data

The data pool contained files from the police which were turned over to the prosecution for final legal evaluation, i.e., to exclude the possibility of a crime. These files—ranging from undetermined causes of disease or death; evident suicides and cases officially relabelled later on as suicides; to undetermined homicide; and accidents in the household and on the job—were analysed by three sociologists with the aid of a coding list comprising eighty variables. The research period covered five years (1981–5). The average number of analysed files per year was approximately 3 800.

Findings

Table 1 shows, on the basis of absolute figures, an average underestimation of official suicide statistics of 25.3 per cent, with a variation between 8.5 per cent in 1981 and 46.4 per cent in 1982. When the two data sources are compared with regard to suicide rates (Table 2), an average increase from 26.7 to 33.5 per 100 000 population, i.e., an under-reporting of 6.8 cases per 100 000 population, is shown.

There is general agreement in the literature that suicide rates are under-reported (Dublin, 1963; Seager and Flood, 1965), but there are only few empirical proofs. Estimates, and there are a lot of them, vary from 25 per cent under-reporting to as much as 50 per cent. Some of these guesses, especially those in the lower range, come numerically close to the results of this study. The under-reporting of 25.3 per cent on an average found in this study represents a considerable amount. Nevertheless, these data were gathered conservatively: one-sixth of 600 missing files, i.e., probably 100 more suicides per year, as well as approximately

TABLE 1: Suicides in West Berlin (1981–5), comparison of official statistics (ICD E 950–9) with research data

Year	*Official statistics*	*Research data*	*Under-reporting*	
	N	*N*	*N*	%
1981	622	675	53	8.5
1982	412	603	191	46.4
1983	490	634	144	29.4
1984	490	613	123	25.1
1985	481	602	121	25.2
Mean	499	625	126	25.3

TABLE 2: Suicides in West Berlin (1981–5), comparison of suicide rates per 100 000 population

Year	*Official statistics*	*Research data*	*Under-estimation*
1981	32.9	35.7	2.8
1982	21.9	32.1	10.2
1983	26.3	34.1	7.8
1984	26.5	33.1	6.6
1985	26.0	32.5	6.5
Average rate	26.7	33.5	6.8

sixty controversial cases per year which appeared to be suicide to the researchers were not included in this study. The under-reporting that was found results from insufficient inter-organisational communication. It is due to the fact that the prosecution fails to inform the bureau of statistics about its relabelling of files from 'death due to undetermined causes' to 'suicides' (which are based, by the way, on *post-mortem* examination in 23.6 per cent of cases).

There has been some controversy about a regulation applied in West Berlin since 1975. This regulation says that if there are doubts about the causes of death the medical coroner should handle these cases as undetermined. Since that time, there has, in fact, been a tremendous rise of the figures representing the ICD category 798 ('sudden death of unknown cause'). Whereas the official figures had been very low during the period before, for example, only seven cases in 1971 and thirty-seven cases in 1975, there was an increase up to an average number of 2 200 between 1981 and 1985. At the same time a gradual decline of official suicide rates took place so that, for example, the difference between the suicide figures for 1975 and 1985 amounts to 75 per cent (Table 3).

In a similar study, Warshauer and Monk (1978) demonstrated that when medical examiners in New York City were given a new option to rule 'undetermined' as a cause of death under the revised eighth ICD, the suicide rate dropped dramatically, i.e., to 66 per cent for Blacks and 50 per cent for Whites. These findings make it evident that a closer approximation to the true incidence of suicide needs to take into consideration not only the official suicide data but in addition the data on undetermined deaths according to the ICD category 798, or—as Barraclough (1973) did—according to the ICD categories E 980–9 (injury undetermined

TABLE 3: Official data on 'sudden death of undetermined cause' (ICD-No. 798) related to official suicide data in West Berlin

Year	*ICD-No. 798* *N*	*Offical suicide data* *N*	*Offical suicide data* *rate per 100 000*
1971	7	860	41.0
1975	37	842	42.0
1981	2.095	622	32.9
1982	2.618	412	21.9
1983	2.614	490	26.3
1984	1.687	490	26.4
1985	1.987	481	25.9

TABLE 4: Rate of ICD-No. 798 data in the federal states of West Germany (1981–5)

Federal state	*Average rate per 100 000*
West Berlin	117.8
Hamburg	47.4
Nordrhein-Westfalen	4.0
Bremen	3.2
Schleswig-Holstein	3.0
Rheinland-Pfalz	2.3
Hessen	2.2
Saarland	2.0
Baden-Württemberg	1.9
Niedersachsen	1.1
Bayern	1.0

whether accidentally or purposely inflicted). The crucial point is, however, to what extent such a combination of data is empirically justified. As some critics in West Berlin stress, suicides are hidden in the classification category 798 for political or bureaucratic reasons to cover up a severe social problem (Wiegand, 1987). This can be underlined and documented with regard to West Berlin in so far as it has the highest rate of 'sudden death of undetermined cause' compared with the remaining ten federal states (Länder) of the Federal Republic of Germany. As Table 4 shows, the average rate totals to 117.8 per 100 000 population, and the contrast with the other ten federal states is striking.

If we proceed according to the suggestion of Pescosolido and Mendelsohn (1986) and distinguish among three kinds of errors which may be associated with official statistics (namely, random error, uniform under-reporting, and systematic misreporting), we can identify the methodological status of these research findings. According to these authors, purely random error reduces the accuracy of empirical investigations but it does not bias the results. With uniform under-reporting, all suicides have an equal probability of not being reported, so that the testing of causal or social theories is not jeopardised, although it raises questions about the magnitude of the effects. Systematic misreporting, by contrast, could obfuscate the true relationship between suicide rates and social causation factors, because the probability that a suicide is misreported varies consistently with social construction factors. When looking again at the prosecutional suicide data of this study, the question arises: what are the consequences with regard to comparative analyses? The distribution pattern on 'sudden death of undetermined cause' shown in Table 4 suggests

TABLE 5: Suicide rates per 100 000 in the federal states of West Germany (1981–5), comparison of official suicides with adjusted ICD-No. 798 and suicide data

Federal state	*Suicide* *rate*	*Rank*	*Rank*	*Suicide plus undertermined* *rate*
Hamburg	31.4	1	2	33.2
Bremen	29.9	2	3	31.7
Berlin	26.7	3	1	33.5
Schleswig-Holstein	25.7	4	4	25.9
Niedersachsen	24.0	5	5	24.1
Bayern	21.7	6	6	21.7
Baden-Württemberg	21.5	7	8	21.6
Rheinland-Pfalz	21.5	8	7	21.7
Saarland	19.8	9	9	19.9
Hessen	18.8	10	10	18.9
Nordrhein-Westfalen	17.4	11	11	17.6

$r = 0.96$; $p \leqslant 0.001$

that this is a Berlin-specific effect. Therefore, the meaning of these data is not that the average under reporting of 25.3 per cent can be generalised and taken as a basis for statistical correction of any official suicide data. Instead, the point is to consider this percentage as indicating the fact that there is a hidden suicide transfer rate in category 798 which amounts to 5.7 per cent on average in West Berlin, i.e., 126 out of 2 200 cases of 'sudden death of undetermined cause'. When we take these 5.7 per cent as a basis for recalculating official suicide data, we get the following rates or rank order, as Table 5 shows.

These data reveal a stable pattern, although there is a change in the rank order concerning the first four federal states (West Berlin at the head of the rank order, followed by Hamburg, Bremen, and Schleswig-Holstein). These four federal states, which represent the northern parts of the Federal Republic of Germany, have a traditionally higher suicide rate than the other parts of the country. That this pattern is a stable one is proved by the fact that, even if one adds the total official number for 'sudden death of undetermined cause' to the official suicide rate (which would be a rather far-reaching assumption, of course), one gets nearly the same rank order, with a rank correlation coefficient of 0.94 instead of 0.96, as in the analysis carried out here based on 5.7 per cent of the total number of cases in ICD-category 798. Therefore, we can conclude that here we are dealing with an unsystematic under-reporting error. With this type of error, comparative analysis is still possible, showing that differences in official suicide rates may vary slightly after correction, but that,

Suicides in West Berlin (1981–5)

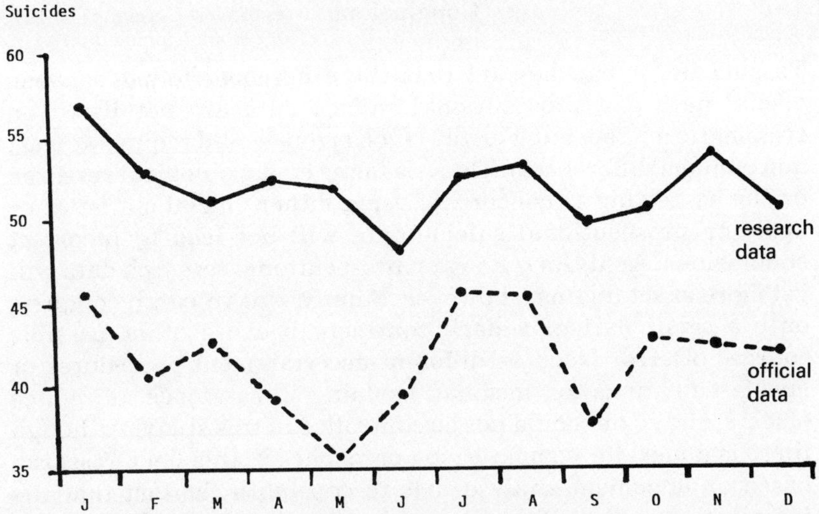

Figure 1: Monthly averages of suicide incidence in West Berlin (1981–5)

in general, such differences reflect truthfully that the incidence of suicide in West Germany does differ from one geographical area to another.

When we finally compare the prosecutional suicide data with the official statistics on a cross-sectional level, we cannot find any statistical differences between the two data pools with regard to global variables. The data for personal status (single, married, widowed, or divorced); for age (classified according to the categories: under thirty years, from thirty to sixty years, and over sixty years); for sex, religion, or nationality, or for the variables 'suicide *modus operandi*' or 'seasonal variation' do not differ significantly. As to monthly suicide variations, Figure 1 reveals a similar curve, apart from the large gap in May. Whereas in other studies (Massing and Angermeyer, 1985; Meares *et al.*, 1981; Näyha, 1982) a peak in spring for instance and cyclic variations of suicide incidence are revealed, the data of this study do not differ from random variation. This might be due to the fact that a research period of five years is too short for a detailed analysis, although one can argue—if cyclic variations are not ecological correlation fallacies (Robinson, 1950) but true phenomena—that they should occur even during shorter time periods.

Conclusions

To sum up, it can be said that the differences found between official data and prosecutional suicide data are not based on systematic misreporting errors (such errors would require at least non-random differences). Thus, as far as epidemiological research or theory testing is concerned, using either official statistics or applying prosecutional suicide data will not lead to incorrect conclusions. Analysts relying on prosecutional research data will get more exact findings, however. Finally, this research conquers only a small part of a dark continent because other possible sources of error (such as different ascertainment procedures or misclassifications of medical examiners, caseloads of police officers, and so on) could not be controlled in this study. Although there is a need for comparative approaches in this field, research based on document analyses has to cope with the fact that the information quality of the files is biased and variable. For various reasons, there is little interest in investigating and handling suicides organisationally or medico-legally like crimes, but this would probably be the only way to improve considerably the information basis for measuring the incidence of suicide more exactly.

References

Barraclough, B. (1973). 'Differences between National Suicide Rates', *British Journal of Psychiatry*, 122, 95–6.

Dublin, L. (1963). *Suicide: A Sociological and Statistical Study*, New York: Ronald Press.

Massing, W. and Angermeyer, M. (1985). 'The Monthly and Weekly Distribution of Suicide', *Social Science and Medicine*, 21, 433–41.

Meares, R., Mendelsohn, F. and Milgrom-Friedman, J. (1981). 'A Sex Difference in the Seasonal Variation of Suicide Rate: A Single Cycle for Men, Two Cycles for Women', *British Journal of Psychiatry*, 138, 321–5.

Näyha, S. (1982). 'Autumn Incidence of Suicides Re-examined: Data from Finland by Sex, Age and Occupation', *British Journal of Psychiatry*, 141, 512–17.

Pescosolido, B. and Mendelsohn, R. (1986). 'Social Causation or Social Construction of Suicide? An Investigation into the Social Organization of Official Rates', *American Sociological Review*, 51, 80–101.

Robinson, W. (1950). 'Ecological Correlation and the Behavior of Individuals', *American Sociological Review*, 15, 351–7.

Rose, K.D. and Rosow, I. (1982). 'Physicians Who Kill Themselves', in S. Shortt (ed.), *Psychiatric Illness in Physicians*, Springfield: Charles Press.

Seger, C.P. and Flood, R.A. (1965). 'Suicide in Bristol', *British Journal of Psychiatry*, 111, 919–32.

Steppacher, R. and Mausner, J. (1974). 'Suicide in Male and Female Physicians', *Journal of the American Medical Association*, 228, 323–8.
Warshauer, M.E. and Monk, M. (1978). 'Problems in Suicide Statistics for Whites and Blacks', *American Journal of Public Health*, 68, 383–8.
Wiegand, A. (1987). 'Rückgang der Todesfälle durch Suizid in Berlin—das Ergebnis einer statistischen Fehlerfassung', *Suizidprophylaxe*, 14, 199–224.

Index

Note: Page references in italics indicate tables and figures.